Feel Fabulous Over Fifty

Feel Fabulous Over Fifty

Gloria Hunniford and Jan de Vries

Hodder & Stoughton
LONDON SYDNEY AUCKLAND

First published in Great Britain in 2000

10 9 8 7 6 5 4 3 2 1

British Library Cataloguing in Publication Data
A record for this book is available from the British Library

ISBN 0 340 74594 0

Typeset by Avon Dataset Ltd, Bidford-on-Avon, Warks

Printed and bound in Great Britain by
The Guernsey Press Co. Ltd, Channel Isles

Hodder & Stoughton Ltd
A Division of Hodder Headline
338 Euston Road
London NW1 3BH

Contents

Preface vii

1 How do I look? 1
2 How do I feel? 7
3 How do I begin to make changes? 13
4 How do I eat and drink healthily? 21
5 How do I know which are the best vitamins, minerals and trace elements? 38
6 How do I look after my weight? 59
7 How do I exercise? 72
8 How do I look after my heart and circulation? 97
9 How do I care for my skin and hair? 116
10 How do I cope with the menopause? 130
11 How do I stave off osteoporosis? 151
12 How do I cope with insomnia? 157
13 How do I care for my partner? 169
14 How do I keep my love life going? 180
15 How do I keep my brain active in retirement? 189
16 How do I get the best out of life? 204

Suppliers 209
Bibliography 211

Preface

It is medical reality that we, as a race, are living longer. In Roman times, the average lifespan was twenty-two years; now the prediction is that in this new century we may expect to work into our eighties and live to well over a hundred. In this book, you may be glad to hear that we are not going to deal with quality of life over the age of a hundred, but will concentrate on the quality of life over fifty. In feeling fabulous over fifty, the emphasis must be on *Energy* and *Vitality* in order to have the quality of life to do all the things we want to in this last third of our lives, whether as part of work or recreation – in other words, to live longer, look better and feel healthier. In the following chapters, we will deal with everything from the A to Z of vitamins, their use and what they do, to the menopause, how to get the best out of life and indeed how to keep your love life active!

I am convinced there is no better person to write this book with than Jan de Vries. He has been a total inspiration to me, and my whole family live by his philosophies and treatments. That's not to say that these take the place of orthodox medicine. Everything Jan talks about is complementary and not alternative.

I first met Jan in 1982 when I arrived in London from Northern Ireland to front a two-hour daily programme on BBC Radio 2. The programme was a mix of music and conversation, and once a month for the following fourteen years, Jan would join me live on air to deal with the nation's queries and questions on general health. To this day, we still broadcast together on my daily television programme *Open House*, in which Jan continues to answer those live questions. I can honestly say that, out of all the experts whom I have interviewed over the years, it is usually melt-down time on the telephones when Jan is on: one particular broadcast on the menopause brought a response of eight thousand letters.

Jan runs clinics all over Britain and I am sure that by the time you get to the end of this book, you too will have decided to make some very significant changes to your attitudes and life, so that you can increase your strength and stamina and *Feel Fabulous over Fifty*.

Gloria Hunniford

1

How do I look?

Imagine the scene at quarter past seven in the morning at London's Victoria Station, where I was waiting for a friend who had kindly offered to take me to a local radio station for an early morning interview. Of the hundreds of people who were passing through the station, my eyes were particularly drawn to those who were obviously taking an interest in their looks. Some were combing their hair, others applying lipstick, still more bringing brushes or mirrors out of their handbags. It was really quite surprising to note how many of these people were taking the time to pay attention to themselves and to their appearance at such an early hour of the day. Others, however, were munching away at a bar of chocolate or an equally unhealthy looking doughnut or pastry.

While I was contemplating these people from all walks of life and of various ages, a lady of around fifty came and sat down close beside me. Out came her beauty case, and she busied herself with applying her make-up. Although I felt that some of her wrinkles might need a fair amount of cosmetics to cover them, the final result was very pleasant. Ten minutes later, to my great surprise, a gentleman appeared, looking equally well groomed. The two fell into each other's arms like two teenagers meeting after a long absence, a passionate scene that also drew the attention of a number of passers-by.

It was at this point that my thoughts drifted to the highly attractive Gloria Hunniford and our work together. I thought of the hundreds of people who had listened to us on Radio 2 when, from 1984 to 1994, I worked monthly with Gloria on her radio programme. Over this long period I also undertook several other radio and television interviews with her, and our working relationship has now progressed to my appearing with Gloria on a regular basis on Channel Five. We have, over the years, answered thousands of questions, on both physical and emotional topics, and I was delighted when, after many requests from listeners and viewers, Gloria agreed to write this long awaited book.

Many of those who wrote in or telephoned remarked on how fabulous Gloria always looked, and wondered what advice I had given her. In fact, I make very little personal contribution to Gloria's good looks – she is well aware of how to look after herself – but I do know that the main reason for Gloria looking so well and attractive is that she pays attention not only to her external appearance, but also to the person within. After all, when we pay attention to ourselves, the end result can only bring about internal contentment and satisfaction that is reflected externally.

One clue to how to do this comes from an old gardener whom we had many years ago. Of his two strawberry beds, one looked wonderful, and there was a fantastic aroma drifting on the breeze from its ripe and succulent fruits. The other bed, however, looked fairly nondescript, being less colourful and giving off only a faint whiff on the sweet smell usually associated with these delicious berries. The gardener explained that he fed the beds differently and this was why they looked so different. The same can be said of the way in which we look after ourselves. If we eat a lot of poor quality food such as pastries filled with a nasty pink sugar and other additives, we cannot expect a beautiful skin to present to the world. We must remember that whatever we feed ourselves is also feeding our outer appearance. This subject will be discussed further in a later chapter.

I continue to see some of my old patients on a regular basis, and it is interesting to observe that many have maintained their beautiful skins. Their 'secret' is that, although they may be eating very plain food, what they are eating is very healthy. A skin that resembles a dried-out prune is often the result of too much twentieth century food containing various E numbers, too much nicotine and excess alcohol. An overindulgence in these substances often results in a worn, uncared-for appearance – we are what we eat and drink.

A poor diet will certainly not enable you to attain a century: we need food that has life and energy in it. Daily I tell my patients that it is necessary to eat as much fresh, organic and wholesome food as possible. Fruit, vegetables, pulses and seeds play an essential and highly important role in maintaining good health, backed up by supplements if necessary. In my early years of working with Gloria, one of the first people I met when I came to the UK, we brought oil of evening primrose to the attention of many people. This supplement has now become of great importance and benefit. Other important nutritional substances are essential fatty oils from fish and low fat protein foods. Drinking plenty of still water detoxifies the body, and anti-oxidants, even in the form of a simple glass of beetroot juice first thing in the morning, are of benefit.

These topics will be covered in more depth later on, but for now we need to look at the challenge of looking after our bodies and our health properly. By paying attention to diet, exercise and mental attitude, the answer to the question 'How do I look?' will be 'Fabulous!'

One particular lady who came to me for advice shows how all these factors can work together. She had been badly let down and was extremely disappointed with life after discovering that her husband had deceived her. Consequently, she was very angry and bitter. As time went by, she stopped caring about her appearance. She developed dark shadows under her eyes, her skin became wrinkled and her hair lost its lustre and good condition, becoming dry and lifeless. Yet deep down she longed to regain her sparkling eyes and clear skin. A little light, and a flicker of enthusiasm, came into her life when she discovered that another man she liked was interested in her too, and she asked me whether I could help her to regain her vitality and health. Alcohol and nicotine had practically taken over her life and she had abandoned all hopes of a positive future. However, once we commenced treatment and she started to believe that life could once again be good, she regained her positive attitude. We also worked on her diet, and she underwent some cosmetic acupuncture to help to smooth out her wrinkles and crows feet, revitalising her skin and complexion. She began to blossom both internally and externally, and her looks improved. Today she is a very healthy, fit, attractive and happy woman because she feels that she has regained her joy and enthusiasm for life.

There is nothing more grateful than the human body: it will react positively if we take positive action to look after ourselves. At the ten clinics at which I consult, I daily come across people who have lost their looks and their zest for life, in many cases for understandable reasons. It can take a long time to motivate and persuade these people to approach life in a positive manner and I sometimes feel that there is a very poor global attitude to life.

This poor attitude to life may lead us to seek a variety of solutions. During a lecture tour of the United States, I often heard raised the topic of hormone replacement therapy, HRT, more of which later. Women often said that they take HRT because they are led to believe that they are old and 'over the hill' after the age of fifty and that, as a result, men will no longer be interested in them. HRT is thus viewed as a form of protection against wrinkles, crows feet and old age, which is, of course, absolute nonsense! A women past the age of fifty has much to offer. Not only has she gathered a wealth of knowledge and experience of life, but she has also developed her personality and talents, all of which can make her much more attractive to others. The same can be said of men – after all we all enjoy and appreciate intelligent, witty and interesting conversation and company. Although this often seems like a cliché, it is true to say that the person within is what makes us attractive to others.

This was brought home to me very clearly by a multiple sclerosis patient I met. Although she was in a wheelchair, it was clear that she was a very lively and sporty person, determined to enjoy life. She fought with every bone in her body not to become, as she said, 'Old, decrepit and done!' Although she was confined to her wheelchair, she was determined to be seen as an attractive and interesting woman. She cared for her skin and her body by following dietary advice I had given her. Thus, outwardly, she continued to keep her good looks. The terrific combination of her determination, her character and her attractiveness was such that if I hadn't been happily married myself, I could quite easily have fallen for her.

As we can see, it is important that we look after ourselves and help ourselves to optimum health and happiness, looking as good as possible by using the many materials now available to us. There is no need for good health and youthful appearance to fade with age. It is simply a question of making some small changes to enable our lives to remain full of vitality and energy. Armed with a basic knowledge of health and science, it is possible to live to an advanced age and still be full of vitality and energy.

So where do you begin to show your body that you care for it and are prepared to make changes for its benefit? I often reiterate at my lectures that man has three bodies – mental, physical and emotional. If these three bodies are in harmony, you will not only feel well, but also emanate a visible sense of well-being and vitality. Thus, as I have suggested above, to protect your appearance you should not only eat a healthy and sensible diet, but also ensure that you get plenty of rest, adequate exercise and a good night's sleep. The chapters that follow will discuss these topics in more detail.

Is energy, then, the key to good health? I have learned over the years that this is certainly true: one wants not only to look good, of course, but also to feel good. The physical body needs that care. But, to look and feel good, the emotional body needs to be cared for with heart and soul. The heart is not only a physical structure but also an emotional being, controlling the external body as well as the inside, hence its importance. Remember this and you will be surprised at how much you can achieve.

In my book *Inner Harmony*, I have written at great length on the importance of harmonising mind, body and soul. By learning how to cope with – and utilise – life's stresses, the positive attitude that follows will improve your appearance. I have seen people with negative and pessimistic outlooks who, on adopting a positive attitude, became happier and developed much more interesting and attractive personalities and appearances. Sometimes when we look in the mirror and ask the question 'How do I look?', we are disappointed with what we see. Some people believe that they are unable, or may in some cases be unwilling, to bring about positive changes in their lifestyle, but *everyone* can fulfil his or her potential for feeling and looking good by taking positive action.

I am often asked how Gloria manages to continue to look so radiant and vibrant with her busy lifestyle. I can honestly say that in all the years we have worked together, I have never seen her in a bad mood, and she never fails to have a positive attitude and outlook. When I asked her how she achieved this, she told me that it was something she had learned from her mother: always strive to remain positive and optimistic; if you have a problem and have done everything to solve it, leave it alone and the problem will resolve itself.

When I was observing all the commuters at Victoria Station and noticing the many different characteristics and attitudes that they displayed, it made me realise how wonderful life is. We should learn that looking good, and maintaining our health, lies in our own hands. After reading this book, and hopefully following its advice, you will certainly feel more fabulous after fifty than you ever did before!

2

How do I feel?

We all have exceptional days when we say to ourselves, 'Why do I feel so marvellous today?' There are special days when you feel completely in harmony with yourself, as if you can conquer the world, and you wish that every day was like this. On these particular days, you are not only happy within yourself, but often a tremendous help to others. As far as Gloria and myself are concerned, we work better with patients, and our television and radio broadcasts may come over so well that people later say how wonderful the advice was or how much help we gave them. On days like these, patients often tell me that they feel extremely good after their treatment, whether it be acupuncture or osteopathy. I have often asked myself why I find such days so extraordinary. Is it bio-energy? Is it because I have been eating and drinking exactly the right things? Is it because I am mentally more alert? Or is there something beyond the human mind that creates these very special days?

I have been practising acupuncture for many years and have been lucky enough to have studied under some of the world's finest teachers, not only in China, but also in Europe. In acupuncture, needles inserted into the skin stimulate unseen energy channels, transferring an electrical impulse along them. The frequency of this impulse influences the strength of the stimulation exerted on that particular acupuncture point. I have been taught the best positions to put the needles in and also how to influence them. One thing, however, I wasn't taught but had to discover through years of practice, often by coincidence: I have learned that the frequency of energy plays an important role in the treatment of acupuncture.

An example of this concerns a patient with multiple sclerosis, a totally incurable condition, who one day got off her bed and walked. At first it seemed almost a miracle, a coincidence or the effect of some supernatural influence, but I then learned that it was caused by neither the needles, nor the machine, but by the frequency of the impulse involved. The way in which we feel and behave often results from the frequencies of life – those frequencies in the cosmos around us – those natural frequencies within the human body, and how they affect us and influence our energy levels. Thus energising certain parts of the body can make us feel good. It is interesting to note that my successes with acupuncture have often been related to the frequencies of the needles that I have used. Put another way, working on the body's energy fields, sometimes called the Chakras, which are influenced by frequencies or energies, has brought them into harmony. Success with acupuncture can be thus achieved by using the right frequency, bringing into harmony the three bodies – mental, physical and emotional.

So how can we influence our body energies to feel good? I have often said that you cannot create good energy by eating an instant desert or a tin of tomato soup that has never seen a tomato, but you can do it by eating good, lively food. You can also influence body energies by exercising, by inhaling oxygen and by feeding yourself with good thoughts. When you feel depressed or down-hearted, or have some illness or disease, hands-on massage, acupressure, reflexology, aromatherapy, osteopathy or acupuncture can help to achieve this too.

The older I get, the more I learn that ignoring or failing to boost our life frequencies can be very costly in health terms. One lovely lady crippled with arthritis came to me for electro-magnetic therapy, a treatment to restore or redirect internal energy. She felt depressed because the handicap she suffered was preventing her work of helping other people using a range of therapies. Although her arthritis remained after the treatment, she felt fabulous because the treatment had given her relief and restored her internal harmony. The frequency of the treatment was important in finding the right balance in her life energies.

Many years ago, I founded, along with Dr Alfred Vogel, the renowned practitioner of naturopathy and herbal medicine, the very first Nature Cure clinic in Holland. We had not long been open when a doctor who was interested in our work, a Dr Koch, paid us a visit. This well-known man was in his day highly advanced in his knowledge of life frequencies and the world of energy. Despite being still very young and inexperienced, I was interested in what he said, as he suggested that he had only scraped the surface of energy, knowing very little about it, and felt that we needed to try to find out as much as we could.

This remarkable man looked at our head nurse and told her that she had headaches every day. In her surprise, she asked him how he knew. He replied that he could see from her outward appearance that, internally, she had a chronic ear infection. She responded that she felt awful every day and did indeed have a pain in her ear. The doctor then told her that he would leave our clinic at five o'clock and that she was to go to bed; then, between five o'clock and a quarter past five, she would find that her ear would start discharging. Someone was to help her to clean her ear and then she would be fine. The nurse did as she was told and asked me to be there too. By ten past five, she called me in great distress as the whole pillow was covered in pus emerging from her ear. But the abscess had gone, and so had the headaches. And she did, indeed, then begin to feel much better.

I couldn't help puzzling over how the doctor had cured this lady. When I later asked him, he replied that he had worked with energy frequencies, treating an imbalance of energy within the nurse's body, to make the abscess burst. The fact that this had happened, and with such speed and efficacy, showed me how much I was unaware of, and gave me a great interest in this area.

Eight or nine years ago at my clinic in Holland, some patients, especially those with incurable conditions such as muscular dystrophy and multiple sclerosis, showed a dramatic improvement. They changed way beyond my understanding, and I knew it was not due to my treatment. On speaking to the patients, they all told me the same story. They had seen a television programme about a doctor in New Zealand who had achieved some remarkable results using differing electrical frequencies applied to appropriate energy points of the body to bring the body's energy levels back into harmony. I enquired further and discovered that this was a Dr Dennis Brooks, who worked with certain energy fields that seemed to create in the body a feeling of well-being, some people with chronic diseases improving beyond belief. I decided to visit Dr Brooks and was amazed at what I saw: his twelve patients were sitting in a darkened room, all holding a lead attached to a transistor radio in the middle. This is, however, not a treatment to be tried without the direction of a qualified therapist. Dr Brooks also used colour therapy, which is now becoming increasingly popular. He kindly gave me all the essential information on his technique, and when I returned a week later to discover that he had died, I was very aware of the significance of my findings.

When I returned to Britain, I enlisted the help of some scientific friends to develop a sophisticated electro-magnetic therapy machine, along the lines that Dr Brooks had used to restore and rebalance the body's energy levels. We researched this and took it to a neurologist in one of the UK's leading hospitals to find out whether a certain frequency might have particular effects. Was there a frequency that would destroy some viruses, for example? The success with the treatment has been phenomenal especially with skin problems, leaving patients feeling much better.

I investigated this further and found that there was still a missing link in the colours that could be used to influence the effect of the frequencies; as I had worked with Dr Ott in the USA, I also believed that it would be beneficial to work colour into the system. I later discovered that similar systems were running parallel to my own, one in particular working well with my own formulae of diet and remedies for different problems. I have now set up these electro-magnetic light therapies in most of my own clinics, achieving much success.

The importance of magnetic energy is suggested by the fact that the earth itself is a giant magnet with positive and negative poles, and negative will always search for positive. Forces released by the magnetic north pole encircle our Earth, and, as we know, energy affects all living things. We are all based in this electro-magnetic field and no life would exist without it. To think that we are such magnetic generators gives us a feeling of importance, yet we must humbly learn to accept that the more we open ourselves up to cosmic energy, the better these magnetic powers will balance themselves.

We saw clearly during the recent solar eclipse the influence of magnetic forces on humans and animals: I have never encountered such quietness and coldness, one in which even the birds stopped singing and humans were quiet. Moon probes have shown that the Earth has not only an atmosphere, but also an ionosphere surrounding it – different layers in which fine electro-magnetic fields surround our Earth. What happens in the ionosphere influences what takes place in our atmosphere and eventually what happens in our bodies. We need to remember, in all the sensible practices and therapies we use, we are aiming to balance these basic forces, and that, as a result of this, we will feel at our best.

When I worked in China, I was taught that the body is a field of energy and that when the energy is balanced, the whole body will function properly. Man has constantly been searching the universe for a simple and better way to achieve and maintain better health. We have long been aware that our bodies have positive and negative energies. As we have discussed, we have polarity, we have magnetic energy, both positive and negative, but neither is able to open up the flow of electro-magnetic power to the organs. To do this, we have to use the head as our control tower and the neck as the magnetic keyboard to interact with the entire body. It is thus important that we learn to care for these areas. Chiropractice, osteopathy and treatment with electrical frequencies can all be used to rebalance and channel the flow of energy from the head via the neck to the rest of the body. When this energy flow is balanced, we will feel at our best.

When I carry out blood tests, I often see that the patient's lymphatic system is very congested, and this too is an important area to tackle to help us to feel good. Cleaning out the lymphatic system will lead to improved flow, which will help to cleanse the blood of waste material. Our life is in our blood, and we can often see the secret power behind the movement of blood, which is of a magnetic nature. It is therefore very important that we carry out blood cleansing, combined with a healthy diet and exercise and plenty of sleep, to influence positively the life force and to feel good.

But I can hear readers saying 'What has this to do with my *feelings*?' It can be seen from the discussion above that the body is an extension of the Earth. We have within us three fine magnetic fields – the emotional electric energy field, the mental electro-magnetic field and the physical electro-magnetic field – which we have to consider. The flow of body energy is like the two ends of a magnet giving their respective polarities to the human body. Not feeling good is the result of disorganised electric forces. You can help to restore the balance by reflexology, homeopathy, osteopathy, aromatherapy or even empathy. From the effects of these we will come to realise that these forces are there to help us and that we must be in tune with them and balance them. It is important to take time to examine what prevents you personally from feeling good, so that you can attain that wonderful feeling of well-being we have all at some time in our lives experienced.

So how can you start to harmonise the body's energy fields in order to feel good? Feeling good means taking action, recognising the daily stresses and practising the following:

Relax – I have cast my burden
Stretch my arms to catch the bounty that is mine
Inhale the one perfect life. Breathe in beauty
Exhale critical and negative thoughts
Brain exercise – think only constructive thoughts
Eye exercise – see only perfection in others
Ear exercise – listen for the voice of the Innate
Facial exercise – smile, smile, smile
Tongue exercise – speak kindness
Head exercise – broadcast thoughts of love
Leg exercise – walk fearlessly in the path that God directs
Soul exercise – commune with the Innate within.

These simple exercises will point you to all you require: health, wealth and happiness.

3

How do I being to make changes?

So many times after my lectures I hear the question 'How can I change my life? I have been eating and drinking all the wrong things. I have been guilty of eating too much sugar, too much animal fat, drinking too much, smoking too much. I want to make a change before it is too late.' The spirit is very willing, but as the saying goes, the flesh is weak, and all too often, I see tremendously good intentions come to nothing. Those who attempt to implement changes in their lifestyle *will* improve their general health but making radical changes is rarely successful: taking things one step at a time is usually more effective.

'But where do I start? How do I re-energise my body? How do I revitalise my life?' The answers to these questions are actually quite clear; putting them into practice is the difficult part. Just ask yourself a few questions: 'Do I really feel up to it, or do I feel tired and exhausted at the end of the day? Do I really enjoy my work or is it a millstone round my neck? Have I really got the relationship with my partner that I want? Is my diet healthy enough? Do I have enough outdoor exercise? Do I have the entertainment I need?'

Are you guilty of the three S's in life – sugar, salt and stress. If so, your body really needs building up. Can you recognise the stresses in your life? Do you drink alcohol regularly? Do you really want to make the changes that are necessary for that fabulous life that you really want – why *not* drink herbal tea instead of the many cups of tea and coffee? If you think along these lines, you will find that there is tremendous room for improvement. Variety is, of course, also necessary. Chapter 4 will suggest how to make simple but effective and varied dietary changes.

There are more questions to ask, too. Is your skin still in good condition? Is your complexion clear? Is your blood pressure a healthy one? Do you feel good? Does your body need reshaping? Have you still got the libido that is necessary for a good sexual relationship? Is your memory as good as it should be? If the answer to any of these questions is no, there is still time to make a change for the better. You have to ask yourself the question, 'Am I more at risk healthwise now that I am fifty? – or have you learnt the lessons of life?

Start by detoxifying your system: as the naturopath Dr Vogel used to say, 'You ought to have a spring and autumn cleanse, like you would your house.' The Detox Box from Dr Vogel (available from chemists and health food stores), which I have prescribed for many years, has been a tremendous help for many. This package contains herbal and homeopathic remedies that will cleanse the body of toxins and waste materials, detoxifying all the body's systems. Another alternative detoxification programme is called Daily Choice Antioxidant, available from the company Enzymatic Therapy. As antioxidants are beneficial in removing harmful free radicals from the body, this will start the change towards a good, healthy life.

Boost yourself and your brain power too. Try Brain Nutrition – a remedy containing vitamins, minerals and trace elements – or, if your mood is low, Mood Food; both these supplements hail from America but are now available in the UK from the company Bioforce. Read a page in a book and test yourself to see whether you can remember every word you have read. If not, read it again and again to exercise your mind. Get into the habit of doing crosswords or playing bridge to stretch yourself, or exercise your brain by joining a class or club.

As you will have a fabulous feeling that life is so much more important now that you are over fifty, change to healthy food that has life in it. Ask yourself whether you have enough fruit and vegetables in your diet: the more the better and eat as much as you can raw. Look at how much animal fat you eat and try to substitute it with vegetable fats and oils. Make sure you get enough exercise and relaxation and a good night's sleep, and that you do not indulge in alcohol or nicotine. Later chapters will give you some tips here.

Lifestyle changes are however not just about diet and exercise – be it mental or physical. You should also get yourself psychologically in order, thinking and feeling positive. Why not do some relaxation exercises, yoga or swimming, walking or cycling? Perhaps have a massage or visit a good health club.

Visualise yourself as the person you want to be – a happy partner, parent or grandparent. I still remember my grandmother at the age of ninety, dancing and singing, telling us that music was the best thing in life, better than any cream cake or drink. Like her, keep yourself happy and positive. A later chapter will give more detail on this. Take a few minutes every day to run through in your mind the negatives that prevent you being happy; see what is there that will stop you feeling totally content. And when you feel sad or neglected, remember that you are an equal human being who has the same rights to life as everyone else. Work on your three bodies – physical, mental and emotional – positively and tell yourself how wonderful you are. Your body will believe what your mind tells it.

Take regular breaks and commune with nature. It doesn't cost anything to go for a walk, absorb cosmic energy and communicate with creation. Even the sound of a bird singing or the sight of some sheep in a field can make you feel good; remember that you too are part of this great creation.

Spoil yourself. Treat yourself with aromatherapy or electro-magnetic light therapy, for example. Think about all the wonderful times that you had in your youth, perhaps how you used to play as a child, and look at the wonderful opportunities that there are for you now. Do things you want to do and do not forget that life is sweet. Remember, however, that it can be too short, so make the most of it and make the changes to benefit you. Your body has been made to enjoy life, and you have wonderful healing powers within you to enable you to make the most of it.

Tiredness is often a major problem, and too many people today suffer chronic fatigue, spoiling their enjoyment of their lives. When emotional conflicts are draining your energies, look for some help: there are some wonderful remedies to give you a life, such as eleutherococcus (Siberian ginseng) to be taken in a dose of 15 drops twice a day. For women, Female Essence, a wonderful combination flower essence available from health food shops, will also give you the energy you need. Allow yourself to take some time and space to think about your problems and what you can do to solve them – only by knowing what to change can we begin to make changes.

There are outside stresses that may hinder you in making changes, for example being the breadwinner or the head of a one parent family. Ask yourself how much stress you feel. If it is family stress, where can you find help? If you have just gone through a divorce and you feel it has messed up your life, look for guidance and counselling, and do not let your problems suffocate you.

I was once visited by a woman who sat down and could not speak. She looked at me and seethed with anger and jealousy. I gave her heather, a flower remedy that is very useful for overcoming jealousy, and listened to her story. She thought that her husband had been having an affair with his secretary, so I went over the facts to see what evidence there might be. At first, she could not speak, but it turned out that the problems were based on unfounded jealousy, and once this factor was under control, she realised that her husband was probably not seeing someone else. The woman had blown the situation up in her own mind so much that they had started to consider divorce. Once this woman discussed the problems with her husband, they made some adjustments to their lives and are now very happy.

One lesson from this story is that when we come to the crux of a problem, we need to spend time looking at the possibilities before we make drastic changes and hurried decisions. There are positive changes and negative changes that we can make in life, but we have to be careful that any changes we make are *carefully* considered. Sometimes it is helpful to neglect a problem for a little while to see whether it will work itself out before we make a change that we may later regret. I have seen patients who have almost come to the end of the road, often because of a lack of communication. It is important that we take time and space for ourselves, perhaps go out for a meal together and talk through problems. Communication can help us to understand our troubles and keep them in perspective.

Family life and financial difficulties can cause many problems. We have all experienced some of these, and we also know that it does not help to moan; we have to take action to solve them. Work often causes problems too. If we work with computers or typewriters, or even if we watch too much television, we need to compensate. Many people have fallen victim to technologically induced illnesses and need treatment to help make the change that is necessary to live life to the full. Stress, resentment or misunderstandings erode our longer life expectancy, and some burdens become too heavy to bear, although it should be remembered that a certain amount of positive stress can be beneficial in sorting out the problem. If there are major changes to be made it is helpful to look at lifestyle, financial status, a person's job and the stress involved. But problems can sometimes disappear, so you should not waste an excessive amount of time and energy worrying – this in itself will harm your health.

Women are subject to their own particular set of difficulties. Many women nowadays experience problems caused by the menopause – the change of life. If, because of the menopause, you have become addicted to nicotine or alcohol to relax, now is the time to stop. There are many ways in which you can give these up if you have difficulty – by acupuncture or rational thinking for example. The menopause may bring with it physical changes as a result of osteoporosis, described in a later chapter, so follow a healthy diet and stay active. Help your calcium levels with good food and remedies such as Urticalcin, five tablets twice a day, which are of benefit for broken bones too.

In domestic life, women can have many burdens, often underestimated by men, so women have the right to look after themselves and tell their partner that help and comfort are needed to cope with the emotional stress, depression, agitation, irritability, mood swings or outbursts of anger brought on by hormonal fluctuations and the stress of their daily lives.

I have a great friend in Canada, Dr Caroline de Marco, who has written a book for women called *The Charge of Your Body*, one of the best books I have ever read. She writes that it is important to analyse your life and figure out the possible sources of stress. She also emphasises the importance of learning to say no, getting help when needed and arranging private time for yourself. Try relaxation techniques – yoga, meditation, aromatherapy massage, a facial or a walk in the country. Acupuncture, osteopathy and naturopathy, for example, may also help to improve your feeling of well-being.

Drinking is another serious problem in today's society, one which can affect men and women alike. I recently saw a couple who were very concerned about their drinking habits. Alcohol had taken over their lives, and they had little money left to finance their habit. We talked about how they had reached this situation. The man had difficulties at work, was underestimated and was bored with the daily routine of a job that he did not enjoy; drink was a temporary answer. His partner had just started the menopause and was trying to suppress her feelings, hiding them from her partner, who was already under so much stress. So she started drinking with him. By now, both were becoming desperate: money was tight, their health was badly affected, and their lives were miserable. A change was necessary.

Even after forty years of experience, I was unable to help them unless they helped themselves. We sat down and sensibly discussed their problems and the alcohol abuse that was affecting their life together. One solution involved teaching the man to appreciate nature, and he was then able to gain satisfaction from getting his garden under control. For her, talking about her opportunities at home and at work gave her the help she needed. By using a variety of herbal remedies and acupuncture, the addiction that she had created was overcome. The negative emotions went and she became happier; she began to feel that she was a woman rather than an alcoholic.

Overcoming a drink problem can be very difficult. Some people do not want to make changes because they derive enjoyment from drinking. Others feel that they want to die and can no longer be bothered. Life has become too much for them and they do not see any need to make changes. It is sometimes very difficult to make these people acknowledge what they are doing to themselves, and to convince them that there is more to life than drink. Drink is only a temporary solution to their distress.

We can all point to some of the reasons underlying certain addictions, be they of alcohol, nicotine or chocolate. Similarly, we all know that addictions have to be overcome and we know how weak we are, but we have to make changes. I have the greatest sympathy for an alcoholic, or those with any other addiction as I myself had to give up coffee to keep my blood pressure in order. Another punishment came when I could no longer eat cheese because it was bad for my heart. Then, when I became diabetic, I had to give up sugar – and here I really struggled. I will be very honest and say that when I see chocolate I have the greatest difficulty in abstaining. Common sense tells me that it is wrong but as we said above, the spirit is willing but the flesh is weak.

But why do I have such a problem with this area? There is an answer underlying every problem, and the reason often has to be discovered in order for a change to be made. My reason is this. As a young boy – on 17 April 1945 – when the Canadian and Scottish soldiers had freed us from occupied Holland, I saw the first chocolate I had ever seen in my life. I went to my mother and showed it to her. She looked at it, broke it into four pieces, gave me a tiny piece and told me to try it. I had never tasted anything so wonderful in my life. Then my mother told me to respect it all my life. It thus became fixed in my mind that chocolate was something that I really should not have. We are all like this; we all want things we cannot have, and forbidden fruits are always those most desired.

Becoming strong and being victorious over the things that we should not have or do gives a wonderful feeling of triumph, not over another enemy, but over ourselves. This is a far greater achievement than any other. Thus the changes that we have to make in life may be difficult but are nevertheless very worthwhile in order to live life to the full. Enjoying those days when you really feel good and in harmony with life, but also in control, is a tremendous victory.

Often when we want to make changes, either at work or at home, we concentrate on the difficulties instead of the positive aspects, which will hold us back. We have to want to overcome the problems we meet, and subconsciously there are experiences stored that can help us to make that change. Once we address our worries and the bad habits that we have developed, we have a goal in life. It is that goal which gives us the determination to make the change. We can do it. Making these changes in life does not need a magic pill: it requires determination to control our own destiny. If we help nature – with positive action, exercise, alternative therapies and little extra treats – nature will help us and make us the people we would like to be.

So take a good look at yourself and your posture. How do you hold your hands, your arms, your feet, your back, your head? What sort of sensations do you have in your muscles, bones and nerves? Do you feel tense and rigid, or do you feel relaxed? Do you see black circles under your eyes? If so, a good kidney cleaner such as Harpagophytum – devil's claw – 15 drops, twice a day before meals, will help more than any cream or make-up. Try now to generate some low-frequency magnetic waves to bring you a sense of calm. Lay your left hand on your forehead and your right hand on the base of your skull. Close your eyes, and breathe through your nose deep into your abdomen. Then breathe out through your mouth. Now you are ready to move on to even greater things. Remember that it is never too late to make a change and that you *can* do it.

I am reminded of the great Nobel Prize winner, Linus Pauling, when at the age of sixty-seven, and at the peak of his career, he thought of retirement. In fact the opposite occurred: from this age to the age of ninety-two, which for some is almost a lifetime, he dedicated his life to helping those around him. After reading a simple little book on vitamin C, which explained how it helped to cleanse the body and enable it to fight infection, he became involved with cancer patients and spent the rest of his life in service to others. By being sympathetic and helping others in their need, he was rewarded with a completely new life. We can all achieve this. It should be not 'Life begins at forty' but 'Life begins at fifty'. The second half of our life, with all the experience that we have gained in the first half, will then be a happy and healthy one.

4

How do I eat and drink healthily?

Maintaining the best possible level of health and preventing the onset of illness and disease is a responsibility that everyone should take upon himself or herself. If an individual chooses to smoke, drink and eat unhealthy and toxic substances, it is useless for them to deny the potential dangers by comforting themselves with the thought that their grandfather or grandmother did just the same. We cannot deny that in today's society, in which our immune systems are so much weaker and more susceptible to environmental pollutants than were those of previous generations, diet becomes an increasingly important factor in preventing and treating illness and disease and helping us to 'feel fabulous'.

When I was involved recently in a radio discussion regarding cancer therapy, one doctor who was very interested in cancer treatment mentioned that it had been proved that 30–40 per cent of cases of cancer could be attributed to an unhealthy diet. I would suggest that this figure should be a little higher as, over the years, I have seen diet play an enormous role in the treatment of cancer.

So what are the principles to be followed for a healthy diet, one which will contribute to all areas of life, as shown by reading the chapters that follow? Each chapter will provide information more specific to that topic, but here I am going to discuss the general approach to eating and drinking for health.

Today I enjoyed a wonderful Sunday lunch cooked by my wife. After the meal, I complimented my wife on how delicious the food had been. She told me that everything I had eaten was organic. Although I am often invited to elaborate dinners, I maintain that there is nothing better than a meal prepared from fresh, organic ingredients. The sumptuous taste and smell of the produce lingers on after the meal has been consumed, and our bodies will soon show the benefits of eating plenty of fresh and organic food containing the vitamins, minerals and trace elements needed (see the chapter describing these) to support our health.

An example will help to explain why this is so important. The last time I was in Teufen, Switzerland, where Dr Vogel and I started our small clinic forty years ago, I returned to a plot of ground where he had at that time planted two cherry trees. They were planted in the same plot, and the trees were of the same origin. Dr Vogel told me that he wanted to grow one of the trees with artificial fertiliser and the other in organic soil. One tree was sprayed with pesticides, herbicides and artificial fertilisers. The other was left to grow and develop under organic and naturally occurring conditions. Dr Vogel asked a very conscientious lady who worked for him to attend to the trees daily, following his exact instructions. She did so, and when I returned to Teufen I went to see the trees. Cherry trees don't normally have a long lifespan, often developing cancerous diseases. The tree grown under artificial conditions had gone, but the other one was still there.

At the beginning of their life, the cherries on the 'artificial' tree certainly looked nicer. However, like much of the produce that we consume nowadays, they had very little smell and taste. In today's society, it is becoming evident that we should return to more organic means of producing our food; we have to take a step back and examine how we look after ourselves.

When I look at those who continue to look young and feel fabulous after the age of fifty, it is obvious that they have looked after themselves. In fact, many of these people eat organic produce and follow a wholesome and sensible diet. These people continue to blossom, and I cannot help but compare their continued good health and vitality to that of the one remaining cherry tree in Teufen. The tree undoubtedly sends forth a message that a natural and healthy lifestyle will continue to benefit and protect the body from the advances of old age and disease.

In the USA each year, over 1.2 billion pounds of pesticides and herbicides are sprayed or added to crops, roughly ten pounds of pesticides for each man, woman and child. Although the pesticides are designed to affect insects and other pests, experts estimate that only 2 per cent of the pesticide actually serves its purpose while over 98 per cent is absorbed into the air, water, soil or food supply. Most pesticides in use are synthetic chemicals of questionable safety. For example, one of the most important environmental factors suggested to play a major role in breast cancer is pesticide residues. Widespread environmental contamination has occurred within a group of compounds known as halogenated hydrocarbons. Included in this group are the toxic pesticides DDT, DDE, PCB, PCP, dieldrin and chlordane, molecules that are hard to break down and are stored in fat cells.

These compounds have been shown to suppress immune function, possess oestrogenic activity and alter hormone levels, all of which could lead to breast cancer. If the levels of pesticides and pollutants in the fat cells of the breast are measured, the results appear to indicate that there is a very strong association between pesticide levels in breast tissue and the risk of developing breast cancer. These results alone make a strong case for choosing organically grown foods. Protection and prevention are obviously better than cure, and in some of the clinics that I have visited, I have seen treatments consisting of organic diet alone, the results of which have been very impressive. It is evident that if we eat and drink healthily, we will reap the benefits of good health.

It is important to increase the amount of fresh fruit and vegetables that we eat, and a highly convenient, effective and tasty way to do this is by juicing. Gloria describes here the theory behind juicing and some of her favourite recipes.

I was introduced to juicing through my daughter Caron. At first, I thought she was just talking about one of those new-fangled and glitzy looking squeezers – but no, she meant a proper juicer through which one can feed fruit and vegetables, skin and all. Caron kept referring to 'The Juiceman' and his theories, and in time, we learned from her to make wonderful mixtures of all sorts of fruit and vegetables, which are a great kick start to the day. Being someone who eats on the run most of the time, I always feel that at least through juicing, I am getting more fruit and veg than I could ever *eat* each day.

When I was in America a few years ago, I finally discovered who 'The Juiceman' was – Jay Kordich, a man who has put forty years into talking to people about these juices, about raw foods, and about how to build a healthy sound body, so that one does not age prematurely. Fruits are often referred to as gods' foods, cooked not by man but by the sun, and full of energy.

Jay Kordich's theory is this: whereas the fibre in all the food we eat is absolutely essential for exercising the gums, helping salivation, keeping the bowels moving and cleansing the colon, it is the juice locked inside the fibre that has to be released. It is the *juice* of the fibre that *feeds* you. Not a speck of the fibre itself, not even fibre that is thinner than a hair, can permeate through the intestinal wall and get into the bloodstream to feed you; only the *juice* is able to penetrate through the intestinal wall, into the liver, to reach the bloodstream and in turn reach every one of your trillions of cells. When you *eat* the food, the body has to process it; all the body is then doing is breaking as much as it can down, so that when your body is digesting the food, it is acting as nothing more than a juice extractor. Why then waste so much of the body's energy breaking down and digesting the food when you can drink the juices themselves, which can get into the system within minutes.

But why should we get our vitamins and minerals from *raw* vegetables and fruits in preference to any other way? Nutritionists are always telling us that the more fruit and vegetables we have daily, the healthier we will be. The answer is because the body's enzymes, protein substances that speed up the body's chemical reactions, are produced by the glands from food elements that may be destroyed when food is heated, as in cooking. We need much live, raw food daily – food containing enzymes themselves – in order to supply the glands with a reserve of these essential and vital substances.

Enzymes themselves are very delicate. They are destroyed by heat, although not by freezing, and they are so delicate that they begin to be destroyed at only 37°C (102°F), being totally destroyed by the time they reach 52°C (125°F). So one could come to the conclusion that when all these enzymes are destroyed, you have 'dead' food – or cooked food. Now the body has to produce these enzymes itself, thus burdening itself with yet another job. It therefore begins to make sense that the more fresh food we eat the better.

The next question is 'Why juices?' Why not just eat the raw vegetables? For *optimum* health, you need more fruit and vegetables than the average person could eat daily. The stomach just cannot cope with that much bulk because the power to break the cellular structure of raw vegetables and absorb the precious elements contained within, is fractional even in the healthiest person. The typical adult absorbs roughly 10 per cent of the value of the food they eat in the form of fruit and vegetables. In the form of juice, however, modern research shows that up to 92 per cent of the elements can be absorbed.

Jay Kordich explains the importance of juices in the following way: the juice of the plant, like the blood in the body, contains all the elements that build and nourish. It's a well-established fact that many of the elements of the plant can be obtained by eating the animal that lives on the plant, that is, if we eat the glandular part of the animal in which these precious food elements are stored, but that means we are getting the minerals and vitamins and enzymes *second-hand* . . . why not eat the plant that builds the body structure of the animal? Raw fruit and vegetables enable us to get our vital elements unspoilt in their entirety. Needless to say, organic produce is best.

Some readers may at this stage be saying, 'I can't be bothered with all that preparing fruit and so on; I'll just buy pre-made juices.' But it should be remembered that everything stored in a bottle or can has been put through a high-temperature sterilising or pasteurising procedure to give these canned and bottled goods a longer shelf-life. On top of that, many juices contain additives and preservatives, and even the tin is treated with chemicals so that its metal will not rust in the juice solution.

There is a wide selection of juicers on the market, complete with ideas on juicing and combinations to try. My first not very expensive juicer lasted for ages before I gave it to my son as a gentle hint to juice for himself. I have now progressed to a slightly more 'industrial' model, but I think that stage only comes when one realises the benefit of drinking these juices regularly.

Here are a few ideas for juices that our family likes. Preparing the juices does take a little while, but we have a rule that the one who washes and prepares the fruit and veg, and does the juicing, doesn't wash up!

For breakfast, pineapple juice is a favourite. Pineapples contain an enzyme called bromelain; apart from containing calcium, magnesium, phosphorus, potassium, sodium, iron and zinc, they are apparently wonderful for taking the pain and swelling out of joints. Just remove the spiny bits on the outside of the pineapple, but juice all the rest, cutting it into chunks that will fit down the tube going into the juicer: if we eat only what we regard as the fleshy part of the fruit, we are getting only a small percentage of the total food value.

Pineapple is also wonderful in a 50/50 mixture with grapefruit. In the preparation, cut off the outer yellow rind of the grapefruit but leave the pith intact so that you get the entire goodness of the grapefruit. Please note that if you are arthritic, citric fruits such as oranges, lemons and limes are likely to inflame the joints, so grapefruit is the only citric fruit recommended in this case. Pineapple can be mixed with mango or papaya for a touch of luxury.

Melon is the number one fruit for total food value. You may consider juicing the rind as well, which increases the nutritional benefits and makes it a very refreshing and aromatic drink, particularly over the summer months. Melon juice is rich in beta-carotene, folic acid and vitamin C, as well as having small amounts of vitamins B1, B2, B3 and B6. It also provides plenty of the minerals calcium, magnesium, phosphorus, potassium and sodium and contains small amounts of copper, iron and zinc. Melon juice should be drunk only on its own. This is because it goes through the digestive system more quickly than any other fruit and would restrict the absorption of nutrients from other juices.

Canteloupe is the queen of the melons as far as content and food value is concerned, rich in beta-carotene to help reduce the risk of cancer.

What we traditionally regard as the edible part of watermelon is a wonderful diuretic, but there are great minerals such as zinc and potassium contained in the white rind and the green shell, probably the number one source of chlorophyll, which is a great cleanser of tissue and a wonderful purifier of the body. These can be released by juicing the whole fruit.

We have all heard the old adage 'An apple a day keeps the doctor away' – with good reason, because apples are representative of some of the best vitamins, minerals, proteins, fats and carbohydrates known in the fruit category. Vitamins A and C ward off colds and flu, the sugar provides a great source of instant energy, and its acid stimulates the flow of saliva. So munching and crunching an apple will start the digestion working properly to break down the carbohydrates in the apple. Apples can be regarded as a kind of neutral fruit in that if you find some of the vegetable drinks, such as carrot or beetroot, a bit strong in flavour, an apple has a neutralising effect; so apples mix with all kinds of fruit and vegetables.

Jan always tells me that the vitamin content of a lemon is much more than that of an orange. Lemons are probably the food richest in bioflavonoids. These substances play a great part in general health and longevity, building up the capillary walls and blood vessels. A lemon drink is wonderful on a daily basis. When juicing, put in the lemon skin, the white membrane, which contains the bioflavonoids, and of course the meaty, juicy part. A quarter of a lemon with about four apples makes great lemonade and is a great diuretic at the same time.

Try the following recipes for fruit juices:

- one apple with 115 g (4 oz) of blackcurrants
- three tangerines and 170 g (6 oz) raspberries
- two large carrots, one stalk of celery and an apple
- ten raspberries together with a small punnet of strawberries
- three apricots and, if liked, 120 ml (4 fl oz) yoghurt

Vegetable juices are particularly rich in minerals and provide an excellent mineral pick-me-up:

- one apple, a quarter of a beetroot and one medium parsnip
- three tomatoes together with a handful of parsley and a quarter of a medium turnip

- two large carrots, six large spinach leaves and a quarter of a beetroot.

Beetroot is a great blood cleanser. Caron makes a point of having it each afternoon, and her children love it too – a wonderful way of making sure that any children you help to look after get enough fruit and vegetables. Caron's mix is beetroot, carrots and apples. For some people, this is a bit of an acquired taste, but the apple helps to diffuse the strong taste of the vegetables.

Although most fruit juices are naturally sweet, you can also add half a teaspoonful of honey, which is of course also very good as an instant pick-me-up.

Many scientists and doctors worldwide believe that when it comes to longevity, the energies, vitalities and vibrations of life are locked in the cells of these sun-baked foods, foods that come out of the ground. Thus, the more fruit and vegetables that you can have raw, the more you will build new cells.

New cells are built through the power of food, and the only food that is live is the raw plant. Remember – it's the juices that are locked in the fibre that feed you.

Proponents of nature cures and nutritional therapy were advocating the use of raw juices long before scientific research had ever thought of investigating them. Now that 'raw juice therapy' has become 'respectable' in the eyes of orthodox medicine, patients are assured of its practicality and are willing to persevere in taking the treatment until the hoped-for results are obtained. It is not surprising that it was in America where these drastic methods of treatment were evolved and practised, as it was there that the greatest crimes against food were committed under the umbrella of 'commercial interests', which subsequently led to disastrous effects on the health of the nation. It was perhaps the prospect of becoming slowly crippled by arthritis that galvanised many sufferers into action and into accepting a raw juice diet rather than face life as an invalid.

It is important to know that patients who have liver and pancreas disorders must not eat stone-fruits such as peaches and apricots in any great quantity as these will probably cause discomfort and pain. Stone-fruit should also never be eaten on an empty stomach. Slow chewing and thorough insalivation of the fruit are necessary. Crisp-bread, rusks and wholegrain bread will diminish the gastric reaction to the hydrocyanic acid the fruit contains. Healthy constitutions used to raw foods can probably digest stone-fruit very well and eat it at any time, but sick or delicate persons should not risk it. If the gastric and intestinal mucous membranes are upset, a tablespoon of clay in water, morning and evening for a few days, will bring relief. Should excessive gastric acidity develop, a teaspoon of wood ash before each meal will help the disturbance.

As more instances of poisons arising from sprayed fruit of all types comes to our attention, we would to well to consider the different aspects of this evil. Some people do not react immediately to poisons such as lead, arsenic, copper sulphate and DDT used in sprays, whereas others are more sensitive and immediately show signs of poisoning. When buying fruit, one should make sure that it hasn't been sprayed. It is common to find blemishes or an occasional brown spot on unsprayed fruit, but this does not affect the properties as far as edibility is concerned. If you are uncertain of whether a fruit has been sprayed, it is better to be cautious and peel it, foregoing the phosphates and other valuable materials that lie immediately under the skin; it is better to do without the minerals, however valuable, than to risk poisoning.

It is to be hoped that such spraying will eventually stop: there is always the possibility of discovering a harmless insecticide that will help to increase crop yield without the risk of harming the consumer. Experiments carried out with herbal sprays, containing extracts of horsetail, yarrow and monkshood, have given very satisfactory results, and investigations into these are continuing. Spraying with tobacco extract is now often recommended as this is much less harmful than chemical sprays.

Berries are very rich in vitamins and should feature far more in our everyday diet. Most of them contain a considerable amount of vitamin C, the importance of which is fully realised in the signs of deficiency, including bleeding gums, the first sign of scurvy, loose teeth, a tendency to chills and a predisposition to haemorrhaging. Allergies and the weariness often felt in spring will be greatly reduced by eating plenty of raw berries.

Blackcurrants are richest in vitamin C, although they have a curious taste that not everybody likes. However, eating 60 g (2 oz) of these daily will provide your body with sufficient vitamin C for 24 hours. Raspberries, redcurrants, cranberries and nearly all other berries are excellent sources of the same vitamin.

Vitamin A is supplied by various other berries: 100 g (3.5 oz) of bilberries contain as much as 1.6 mg of vitamin A. The principal sources of vitamin A among the vegetables are carrots and watercress.

Experience has shown that berries are good for the liver. In pancreatic disturbances, bilberries will do much to restore order, whereas stone-fruit, pears and so on can have a harmful effect. The one berry that has to be watched is the strawberry. Many people are allergic to strawberries, and these can also affect the kidneys, although much depends upon the fertilisers used in their cultivation. If natural manure or compost rich in bone meal and natural lime is used, they may not cause reactions. If you are allergic to cultivated strawberries, try the wild ones because there is a difference.

Patients with lymphatic congestion will frequently have reason to complain of swollen glands, and anyone thus afflicted should make the fullest use possible of all available berries, which may help to reduce their tendency to infectious respiratory diseases. Mothers-to-be in the family may similarly benefit from berries: they may be interested to know that when there are sufficient vitamins (especially vitamin C) and minerals in the blood, most of the ailments associated with pregnancy, including morning sickness, can be avoided.

Fruits and juices can be incorporated into a range of diets, with great results. For many years I had tremendous success with a special diet that Dr Vogel used to recommend to many patients. Not only did I find this alone to be very helpful to the patients, but it was also very beneficial when used in combination with the raw juice of a potato. This special diet is described below. It can be used by anyone at any age to improve general health and relieve many physical complaints. If strictly adhered to, this diet will cure a stomach ulcer within a month, gout or any rheumatic complaint disappearing within two or three months.

Before breakfast, take half a glass of raw potato juice diluted with warm water. Breakfast itself should consist of whole wheat that has been soaked in water for two or three days; this can be made more palatable with the addition of vegetable stock or butter. Crispbread with butter and wheat germ will complete your breakfast. If the bowels need special attention, add psyllium or freshly ground linseed to the wheat. If your liver is not functioning properly, drink a glass of raw carrot juice. Remember to chew all the food thoroughly.

Lunch should be a good, strong vegetable soup with a cup of raw cabbage juice added after the soup has been taken off the heat. This is then followed by a dish of unpolished brown rice, whole wheat, buckwheat or millet, steamed vegetables and a salad. Never use vinegar to make your salad dressing; instead use lemon juice, sour milk or whey concentrate. If you feel nervous and tired, every second day, take a beaten raw egg and add it to your food. On no account should the eggs be cooked because this will destroy most of their vitamins and, in addition, lead to a build-up of uric acid; only raw eggs have a place in a curative diet.

Supper can be along similar lines to breakfast. The whole wheat dish can be varied by taking oat flake porridge or preferably raw, soaked oats, put through the mincer. Instead of fruit, use fruit juices only on this special diet.

Sausages, pork, canned foods, white sugar, white flour and anything made from white flour are to be avoided for the rest of your life. If you must, you may start eating meat again after six months, but only beef or veal. Carry out this diet faithfully and you will find that the most difficult case of gout will disappear.

Natural remedies will, in the majority of cases, hasten any healing process. Never lose sight of the fact that the healing depends fundamentally on the raw juices. As these juices, with the exception of carrot juice, are not very palatable, try mixing them in a soup and adding them just before serving. The juices may be warmed in a double boiler so as not to cool the soup too much, but they must not be boiled. Patients with severe cases of stomach ulcers should drink at least two cups of the juice daily.

As mentioned here, and as Gloria has already described, cooking can destroy the nutritious elements of fresh fruit and vegetables. So where does this leave us in terms of preserved fruits, such as fruit bottled from the garden? During the sterilisation of the fruit – assuming that a natural process is used – the high temperature obviously destroys many of the vitamins, but the actual nutrients, such as carbohydrates, sugar, starch and minerals, remain unchanged. It is, however, quite a different story with commercially preserved fruits and vegetables. Bleaching, shaping and adding chemical preservatives definitely has a direct and negative effect on the food value after processing.

So do sterilise and bottle all the leftovers from your garden produce, but do not make the mistake of depriving yourself of fresh fruits and berries just because you want to preserve them. I remember as a child having to watch the blackcurrants and raspberries I longed to eat being made into jam; parents, in their eagerness to preserve, sometimes forget about the value of fresh fruit.

When making jam, use unrefined brown sugar as white refined sugar is a calcium destroyer. The sugar contained in fruits is, of course, the most valuable of all, and berries are very rich in this. As extra sugar must, however, be used in making jams, it is best to use brown sugar with at least 10–20 per cent grape concentrate added to give it still greater food value.

For the sake of convenience, factory-preserved foods are often used when the meal could, with a little extra effort, incorporate fresh fruits or vegetables instead. Canned foods are used all too often by hospitals and sanatoriums, and this has now become the norm. If sick people are to get well, they must have health-giving nourishment, which can be obtained at its maximum value only in fresh foods. For this reason, one should eat fresh foods as much as possible during harvest time. Eat your vegetables raw in salads as much as you can, and eat fruits and berries by themselves or in muesli or fruit salad. Anything that cannot be used should be sterilised and bottled when fresh so that provision is made for the winter.

It is not necessary for everything you eat to have a high vitamin value; the important thing it to make sure that you do not omit anything essential when planning your menu. Let's suppose that for lunch in the winter you have yoghurt, which contains vitamins, and some fresh carrots, turnips and cabbage salad. To this, you may add preserved vegetables, followed by potatoes or unpolished rice. The body will obtain its vitamins from the fresh vegetables, and its other nourishment from the canned or bottled materials. Thus, you will have ensured all the nutrients you need to keep you feeling fabulous.

While we are on the subject of cooking, we need to consider cooking utensils themselves. Years ago, copper utensils were used to a considerable extent in hotels and restaurants, and were considered a prerequisite in any well-to-do home. With the knowledge we have today, it is easy to do without copper, especially when it is known that it destroys vitamin C. Rose hip purée and barberries (an Australian fruit), for example, are both rich in this vitamin, but if they are prepared in copper kettles, they will lose much of their vitamin value. On the other hand, steel- and enamel-covered pans have no effect on the vitamin content.

In addition, copper oxidises easily and forms verdigris, which may cause poisoning. It has been observed that the use of copper utensils leads to gastroenteritis. The liver may obviously be affected as well because everything assimilated from the digestive tract finds its way directly through the portal blood circulation to this organ. Jaundice, anaemia, damage to the kidneys and minor disturbances in the central nervous system, possibly even Alzheimer's disease, can often be traced to the regular absorption of metallic oxides and salts from copper and aluminium utensils. If the fantastic dilutions of copper used in homeopathy to treat arthritis can affect the body, how much greater must be the effect produced by the physical use of copper utensils in contact with our food.

Aluminium falls into the same category as copper. If we wish to cook health-giving food, we will have to make sure that the pots and pans we use meet proper standards. It is difficult enough to steer our way through the maze of dangers that beset our foods – preservatives, chemical adulterations, sprays, etc. – all of which destroy the nutritional value of our foods, without generally lowering food standards by cooking with utensils that are harmful.

One thing that I strongly advocate is the growing of herbs and shrubs in containers at home. These herbs can be easily added to household meals; for example Salvia (sage) added to the food will help to keep menopausal hot flushes under control. Many garden herbs can be used in many homemade beauty lotions.

One of the most important influences in our diet is our consumption of coffee and tea, which are both easily addictive, tea also containing a high tannin and caffeine content. Therefore, I often recommend my own brand of Health Tea, which is based on my great-grandmother's recipe. Not only is it beneficial for a myriad health problems, as well as assisting in keeping the weight down, but it is also very nutritious. When leading a busy life, many of us tend to reach for a quick cup of tea of coffee. It would be much more beneficial if we drank Bambu coffee or Health Tea. For those wishing to read further on this subject, Dr Vogel talks quite a bit on coffee in his book *The Nature Doctor*.

Millions of tons of coffee are consumed annually. Because of its composition, it is not surprising that many people concerned with their health are discussing it via all sorts of media. Coffee can damage our health, having been shown to have a definitely injurious effect on the nerves. It also adversely affects the skin and blood pressure, and is involved in inflammatory bowel syndrome and other bowel problems. Although I disapprove of the regular use of coffee, even I have drunk coffee on occasions when I needed to stay awake for a long drive at night. If one is not a regular coffee drinker, and only takes it occasionally as a stimulant, its immediate effect is surprising, but if, however, you drink coffee regularly, this is not apparent.

Surprisingly, Arabian coffee can be prepared in a way that is much less harmful than that used in the European or American home, and its stimulating effect is hardly noticeable. The Arabs serve their coffee, as the Turks do, in little cups, along with the grounds. As a rule, Arabs prepare the coffee when the guests arrive, and they never store it once it has been roasted and ground. It is usually served very strong with the grounds and sugar, but in comparison with regular coffee and cream, this drink seems less stimulating. Apparently, the grounds contain certain substances that to a certain extent neutralise the components such as caffeine and also weaken the stimulating properties of the coffee.

It is a matter of choice whether one would rather drink coffee prepared in the Arabian way than destroy its natural flavour by extracting the caffeine, which may not be the most harmful substance, to leave caffeine-free coffee. As other components of the coffee also affect the health adversely many different opinions are encountered on the subject.

To rid the coffee of its caffeine, inorganic substances such as benzol or similar coal tar derivatives are used, which begs the question of whether decaffeinated is really better than regular coffee.

Percolating is not the best way to prepare it as it loses much of its taste and aroma, so one loses out on the quality, obtaining a dark frequently slightly bitter brew. Those who insist on drinking coffee should prepare it by the filter method.

All in all, it seems that the real answer is that most coffee drinkers should give it up completely for the sake of their health; this can easily be done by using a coffee substitute.

Efforts to find a satisfactory substitute for coffee have been going on for over fifty years, with the result that there are good cereal and fruit mixtures on the market today that have many advantages for health and none of the disadvantages of the bean coffee. Aside from the contents, the cereal and fruit coffee, when drunk with milk, is ingested much better, turning into a fine, flaky mixture rather than a lumpy curd in the stomach. For the nervous, sensitive and highly strung people, who should abstain from coffee altogether, cereal coffee is an excellent substitute.

Father Sebastian Kneipp, a pioneer of hydrotherapy, introduced a malt coffee that is still sold today although many other coffee substitutes have since appeared that are in many ways superior. Cereal and fruit coffee enjoys increasing popularity as it offers more health value than malt coffee. The next time you go to the health food store try it. It may take a while to get used to it, but you will then learn to enjoy it, to the benefit of your health.

It is not unreasonable to suggest that if we take the trouble to stick to a healthy diet, this should be accompanied by a good coffee substitute. A confirmed coffee drinker might think that it would be impossible to get used to a substitute; those who feel like this should try adding the cereal and fruit mixture gradually, increasing the amount of this and decreasing the amount of regular coffee until it is made up entirely of cereal and fruit coffee. From then on, the palate will prefer the new substitute and the heart and nerves will benefit tremendously.

As well as knowing which foods are the most beneficial for us to drink and eat, it is also necessary to know how to eliminate toxins and how and when to fast. Further advice on these topics can be found in the book *Nature's Gift of Food*. Most of us tend to consume food containing hidden toxic materials so detoxification of the body is very important. It is essential that constipation is not experienced as the body should eliminate whatever has been consumed within forty-eight hours.

When I carry out blood tests on my patients I am often amazed at the terrific amount of toxic material present in their systems. As a result, I often have to prescribe a strong detoxification formula, such as Doctor's Choice Antioxidant (available from Enzymatic Therapy), which provides fifteen of nature's most powerful anti-oxidants – protectors against damage caused by toxins – in one supplement. One capsule three times daily should be taken as an addition to the everyday diet. The capsules contain, among other things, beta-carotene, vitamin E, vitamin C, selenium, zinc and manganese, all of which have anti-oxidant functions. Procyanidolic oligomers from grape seeds and green tea extract are 50–200 times more potent even than vitamin E, and concentrated extracts of cabbage, garlic, ginger and Klamath blue-green algae are rich dietary sources of anti-oxidant nutrients. The capsules contain no sugar, salt, yeast, wheat, gluten, corn, dairy products, colouring, flavouring or preservatives.

The Blood Detoxification Factors preparation from Michael's, which is also available from Enzymatic Therapy, contains nutrients known to be essential for the proper functioning of the blood detoxification process, such as iron, manganese, zinc, molybdenum, echinacea, red clover, burdock, gotu kola and yellow dock root.

For full health, it is very important to maintain normal bowel tone and ensure its regular function. To help with this, I would recommend a product called Eliminex, derived from an extract of chicory root. It is both non-toxic and non-addictive, with a gentle non-irritant action that helps to maintain regularity and nourish gut mucosal cells. Eliminex works in three ways. First, the chicory extract helps to carry moisture through the digestive system, keeping waste matter soft and bulky, and thus helping to maintain a healthy bowel function.

Secondly, as Eliminex passes through the bowel, it is used as a food substrate by beneficial bacteria such as *Bifidobacterium bifidum* and *Lactobacillus acidophilus*. These bacteria consume the complex carbohydrates in Eliminex and in turn release organic acids into the bowel, thus lowering the pH of the bowel. This suppresses the growth of pathogens such as *Escherichia coli* as well as stimulating peristaltic movements in the bowel wall. Pathogens are further controlled by being 'crowded out' by the beneficial bacteria, the latter multiplying rapidly in response to the food source supplied by Eliminex, which cannot be used by the pathogens.

Finally, the growth of beneficial bacteria provides an energy source for the gut epithelial cells. Many nutritionists believe that maintaining the health of these cells is important for digestive well-being.

Eliminex can be dissolved in a hot or cold drink, or sprinkled directly onto food. Its pleasant taste means that it can easily be added to drinks and foodstuffs without affecting their palatability. Eliminex is suitable for all ages, as well as for diabetics, those on yeast-free diets and those taking medication.

So now we have an idea of which foods to eat and which to avoid, as well as how to detoxify our bodies. In various ways, our bodies forewarn us of their degeneration. If we look carefully at our teeth, our bones and indeed our general state of health, it may appear that people are living longer, but it is the quality rather than the quantity of life that we should be pursuing. Organic food should be the basis of our staple daily diet, on top of which sunshine, water, air, exercise, efficient digestive function and supplementation should also be integrated into our daily pursuit of a healthier lifestyle. It is important to recognise that you are part of creation and that you should respect your body. Feed it with what is necessary and it will continue to support you. The body does not lie but we may not always take time to listen to it. If we learn to be in tune with our bodies, they will tell us exactly what is happening internally, advising us how well they can function and undertake the activity that we demand of them at this special stage of our lives.

5

How do I know which are the best vitamins, minerals and trace elements?

Nowadays, the use of vitamins is widespread and much talked about – even orthodox medical circles are at long last accepting that the use of extra vitamins over and above our daily intake of food, can help in certain conditions. Jan has, for example, been administering oil of evening primrose for forty years, but it is only of late that medical authorities have accepted its healing and helpful qualities.

As for me, for some extraordinary reason, I have been hooked on the idea of vitamin use since I was seventeen though living in semi-rural Northern Ireland, where bottles of vitamin pills were certainly not on my mum's shopping list every week. On reflection, I think that my fascination arose through the movies. There was not much to do in our small market town except going to the pictures. We had three cinemas in Portadown, and as they changed their programme three times a week, we saw a lot of films. Those of you old enough will remember that, in those days, there were many film books and annuals to go along with our matinee idols, which I of course devoured on a daily basis. That celluoid world was our escapism, and I was always totally intrigued, when reading film star biographies. Although they were usually over sixty – which was the end of the road as far as we were concerned – they still looked young and vibrant, and at least twenty years younger than they really were. In my mind, it was definitely the forty or fifty vitamin pills they took daily that did the trick, so, from my early teens, multivitamins were always on my shopping list. My mother was always bemused with the idea; she was a marvellous cook and thought I should not be looking beyond her nurturing meals.

Here, of course, lies the age-old argument concerning vitamins, one which I have been involved in many times on air. Ask any doctor about vitamin use and the verdict is always, 'If you have a properly balanced diet, you don't need any extra vitamins.' I absolutely agree – but show me who nowadays actually *does have* a properly balanced diet, balanced in nutrients and minus all the preservatives, additives and so on. So I have always been, in my own basic way, of the opinion that I should help the natural process along a bit, working a little on the 'just in case syndrome'. Until I met Jan, I consumed just multivitamin preparations, but when I got to know more through him, I arrived at a more planned programme.

Journalists who interview me are always a trifle surprised when I tell them I sometimes consume up to thirty-five tablets a day, depending on my schedule. For example, I always take vitamin C, because Jan tells me that, of all the vitamins, this is the most important, as well as vitamin E, to try to prevent heart disease and to improve my skin. I take extra calcium, too, partly because I had a very bad fracture some years back in my shoulder, and partly, of course, to prevent osteoporosis.

My shoulder injury is a good example of orthodox and complementary medicine working hand in hand. I had broken the ball and socket of my right shoulder into fifteen pieces and fractured my right humerus through a freak fall while playing tennis. It seems crazy such an injury could take place while trying to keep fit, but, I had done something I don't ordinarily do, running to reach a sneaky drop shot. As I ran, my toe caught the indoor felt, and I did one of those staggering and dramatic falls. To cut a long story short, I had to have four operations over three years.

To my surgeon's surprise, the ball and socket mended quite easily but the humerus bone would not knit and he recommended a bone graft from my hip joint. As I could not bear the thought of yet another joint being out of action, I asked for a stay of execution; laughing, he gave me six months' reprieve. So Jan set to work with homeopathic treatments on the tissue and bones, and, to my great delight, by the next X-ray, the arm had mended. Some will say that this was a coincidence, but I was thrilled to avoid a painful bone graft and escape a further operation.

I truly believe that the way forward is a combination of orthodox and complementary medicine with an emphasis on prevention. Augmenting what we eat in our daily lives, taking extra vitamins on an informed and constructive basis, can only be a positive step forward. I still think those old Hollywood stars had it right!

One can read almost every day in newspapers or journals that it has been proved that many people lack vitamins, minerals and trace elements. Daily we see patients who have problems that can be seen to improve when supplementary vitamins, minerals and trace elements are used. Even serious illnesses and degenerative diseases can be greatly helped by good dietary management. It is obvious too that our processed fast-food diets are deficient in many of these essential substances, and pollution, the use of insecticides and the stresses of modern life make it even more likely that we will become deficient in these vital nutrients.

Because of the lack of quality in our factory-grown food, we have to consider supplements, whether multiple or single. We all need different amounts of these: Gloria takes many more vitamins and minerals than I do – but she has a much more stressful life on radio and television, and I am in the lucky position of eating a lot of organic food, which is tremendously helpful.

The vitamins, minerals and trace elements will be described in turn below. Although some of these may be more relevant than others to those over fifty, they have all been included as some readers will undoubtedly care – sometimes or often – for their own children or grandchildren and will want to ensure that they too are as healthy as possible. Taking more than the recommended daily intake of natural vitamins in food does not hurt us, but the same cannot be said of synthetic vitamins. These artificial products should only be taken in accordance with a prescription and are never equal to the vitamins contained in plants or fruits. So if you believe the principle that food should be a medicine, you will not take synthetic vitamins but make sure that your daily requirement comes from carefully chosen and prepared food.

Vitamin A

This vitamin, although more often deficient in infants and small children than in adults, is important because a deficiency leads to conjunctivitis and dehydration of the cornea as well as predisposing one to skin diseases, glandular malfunction leading to obesity, night blindness, lung ailments, pneumonia, inflammation of the middle ear, suppuration, the development of abscesses and so on, as it is important for immune function. So where do we find this important vitamin? It occurs in butter, cod liver oil, dandelion leaves, nettles, parsley, savoy cabbage and, as provitamin A, in carrots. Fruits containing vitamin A are apricots, dates and rose hips. The recommended daily dose is 800 μg.

A vitamin A deficiency can quickly be overcome by taking cod liver oil, rose hip syrup and date sugar. Anyone whose assimilation is poor should take the condensed juice of biologically grown raw spring carrots: Biocarottin, available from most health food shops and taken in a dosage of one teaspoonful daily, has the advantage of being a tonic for the liver. It is unnecessary to buy expensive vitamin preparations when natural foods such as those given above serve the purpose much better.

Carrots are a vital source of vitamin A and so rich in important minerals and vitamins that they can rightly be called a remedial food. You should eat them every day in one form or another – perhaps as salad or freshly prepared raw or juiced – especially during the low-vitamin winter months and early spring. They should preferably be eaten raw, because when uncooked they retain all their goodness. Children like to nibble carrot sticks as if they were sticks of rock or candy – a good tip when providing your own family with a meal. I remember when eating carrots used to mean tucking into a dish of boiled carrots, sliced and buttered, but since the importance of vitamins has become common knowledge, eating grated raw carrots, exceptionally refreshing with a little grated horseradish, has become far more acceptable.

Why, then, are *carrots* so good for us? One kilogram (2.2 lb) of carrots contains approximately 2.5 g potassium, about 300 mg calcium, 6 mg iron and 0.6 mg copper, the latter two substances being important constituents of the blood and better absorbed from plant material. Carrots are also rich in phosphorus, which is helpful for the brain, especially the memory, and also iodine, which is good for glandular function, particularly of the thyroid. Furthermore, carrots are a source of magnesium and cobalt, as well as carotene (provitamin A) which gives rise to vitamin A when it is metabolised.

Carotene is extremely important in our efforts to keep our cellular system healthy and our digestive organs functioning efficiently. It promotes healthy growth and the development of strong, resistant teeth: in fact, vitamin A, together with calcium and vitamin D, contributes considerably to the formation of good teeth.

Did you know that carotene, if taken plentifully, is also able to resist the formation of kidney stones? A lack of carotene contributes to susceptibility to infection, especially coughs and sneezes. In addition, taking the recommended daily intake of carotene helps to achieve a faster and more complete recovery in cases of pneumonia, heart troubles, eczema and psoriasis. As mentioned earlier, it is generally known that it is good for the eyes; it can help to improve eyesight and, if taken in sufficient quantities, can be the means of overcoming night-blindness – a tremendous benefit for pilots and night-drivers. Carotene has another welcome benefit in that it reduces the tendency towards cataracts.

In addition, experiments and observations are said to have shown that carotene improves the function of the sex glands because it exerts an influence on the production of sex hormones; this can be of assistance in overcoming sexual weakness and impotence. This effect may be attributable to the high vitamin E content of carrots. Finally, 1 kg of carrots also contains 0.5 mg of vitamins B1, B2 and B6 as well as vitamin K and about 50 mg of vitamin C, the valuable nerve food. All these vitamins will be described below.

Vitamin E

The Roman gladiators had no idea about hormones and vitamin E, but they knew from experience that they became more energetic and efficient when they ate bulls' testicles the day before their contests. As with many of the discoveries that serve us today in our quest to rectify errors in nutrition that plague us in the form of deficiency diseases and avitaminoses, clear thinking, acute observation and some degree of biological understanding – as well as mere chance – were needed to unravel this mystery.

Vitamin E itself, also known as alpha-tocopherol, was discovered in 1922 by the American scientist Herbert McLean Evans, although it was many years until its functions began to be fully understood. It protects polyunsaturated fats in the diet, such as fish and seed oils, against being oxidised to produce free radicals which damage cell membranes. It is thus known as an anti-oxidant. It does not, however, work alone but has a close relationship with vitamin C and beta-carotene (see vitamin A, described above). It has now been proved that there is no better natural remedy than vitamin E for sterility and infertility – many women could have saved themselves great heartache had they known about vitamin E. Not only does this vitamin prevent miscarriage, but it also promotes the healthy development of the foetus, ensuring a normal pregnancy without complications.

Vitamin E, however, is not only important for women: men too depend upon an adequate supply for normal functioning of sex glands. Since the secretions of the reproductive glands, the hormones, are to a large extent responsible for one's general well-being, vitality, stamina and pleasure in work and achievement, it is obvious that vitamin E, which influences the formation of these hormones, assumes a major role in the maintenance of health.

In addition, vitamin E influences the development and function of the smooth and striated muscles, being able to prevent muscle degeneration, especially important for cardiac (heart) muscle. In fact, vitamin E (in a dose of 500 units twice daily), together with a natural heart remedy such as crataegus (ten drops twice a day), has proved most effective as a tonic for weak heart muscles. Vitamin E is also involved in producing healthy connective tissue, blood vessels and has been recommended as an excellent remedy for burns and poor clotting, as well as in warding off the effects of ageing. Menopausal problems also respond well to average doses of vitamin E, as do rheumatic ailments. As it is involved in the efficient use of oxygen by the body, it is important for all those taking physical exercise.

The correct daily dosage of vitamin E has not yet been established, but it is assumed that the daily requirement is 15–25 mg, which is contained in about 15 ml (about half a fluid ounce) of wheat germ oil.

Vitamin E is not found in meat, except in those parts that are today viewed as unsuitable for human consumption, for example bulls' testicles, spleen, placenta, pancreas and pituitary gland. It is, however, found in fish and egg yolk and in small amounts in milk as well as butter.

It is more abundant in vegetable products, primarily cereal germ, oily fruits and cottonseed, as well as corn (maize), peanuts and all varieties of cress – watercress, garden cress, nasturtium and American cress. For this reason, herbal seasoning salts, Herbamare and Trocomare, which should be used as you would normal table salt, include these cresses. Vitamin E is also present in spinach, lettuce and alfalfa (lucerne), as well as in most leafy greens. Vegetarians usually meet their daily vitamin E requirement more effectively than meat-eaters. If you suffer from a deficiency, make use of these sources.

For quick results take wheat germ oil, or, if you do not like its taste, wheat germ oil capsules, which are quite easy to swallow. Raw wheat germ is the richest source of vitamin E, and this wonderful food has been neglected for too long; in autumn, a dish of berries sweetened with honey and covered in wheat germ should be found on everyone's table.

Lamberts vitamin E capsules present vitamin E in its natural form as d-alpha-tocopherol, which is how it appears in food such as nuts and vegetable oils; it is in the form of d-alpha-tocopherol that vitamin E is most easily absorbed. The vitamin E used in these Lamberts products is naturally sourced, which is much better than using an artificial product.

Vitamin C

In order to see how important it is to prevent vitamin C deficiency, we would do well to refer to Captain Cook's famous experience. Realising the disastrous effect of a lack of vitamin C in the diet, such as sore joints and bleeding gums, and to guarantee the success of his expeditions, he carried on board whole barrels of sauerkraut, his farsightedness sparing him and his crew from falling victim to scurvy. Every 100 g (about 3.5 oz) of sauerkraut contains approximately 20 mg of vitamin C, about the same proportion as in raw potatoes – although the latter are, of course, far less palatable!

The symptoms and consequences of vitamin C deficiency are muscular weakness, bleeding under the skin, bleeding of the gums and loosening of the teeth, which can even fall out. Resistance to infectious diseases is greatly reduced, and susceptibility to catarrh, sore throats and tonsillitis, pneumonia and pleurisy is considerably increased. The capillaries are weakened and damaged, severely affecting the circulation.

Although there is no unanimous opinion regarding the daily requirement of vitamin C, this seems to be between 75 and 100 mg for adults and about half this amount for children, for whom you may be caring. The following list will give you some idea how to cover your daily requirement. The quantity of each food item for this purpose is given in grams (1 g = 0.035 oz; 1 oz = 28 g); for example you would have to eat 12 g of sea buckthorn berries to obtain the amount of vitamin C needed for one day.

- 12 g of sea buckthorn berries or raw sea buckthorn purée
- 20 g of ripe rose hips or raw hip purée
- 70 g of blackcurrants
- 20 g of green cabbage salad
- 170 g of strawberries
- 180 g of spinach salad
- 200 g of white cabbage salad or natural sauerkraut without additives
- 300 g of dandelion salad
- 500 g of potatoes boiled in their skins

The amount of vitamin C contained in each item is only approximate, the actual figure varying according to where the plants grow and the season, but fresh fruits or vegetables have the highest content when freshly picked as a certain amount is lost in storage. It goes without saying that you will only need part of the amount given for each food item containing vitamin C because you will eat more than one category of food in the course of the day. If sugar is added to the raw, freshly prepared fruit purée, a larger amount of fruit will be needed to cover your requirement. To set your mind at rest, I would like to point out that the natural vitamin C in our food does not harm the system, even though we might take in more than the indicated daily quantity. Bio-C Lozenges, made from fruit extracts with a high natural vitamin C content, taken in a dose of three or four daily, are of benefit. These can be obtained from chemists and health food shops.

Vitamin C can also be taken as time-release tablets; these contain ingredients that are formulated in a special mixture retaining the nutrient in micropellets and allowing it to be released slowly after the tablet has been ingested. This means that the absorption of vitamin C is a continuous process as a gradual release takes place over six to eight hours.

The advantages of time-release vitamin C tablets are:

- a gradual release of vitamin C, which copies the natural process of food digestion
- a more even level of vitamin C in the blood for a longer period
- a slower rate of excretion of vitamin C
- the beneficial effects of vitamin C being available over a sustained period.

Lamberts Time Release formulae also supply bioflavonoids, which are organic substances that accompany vitamin C wherever it is present in fruit and vegetables. These bioflavonoids appear to assist in the optimum absorption and use of vitamin C and help to maintain the integrity of the blood vessels.

Time-release vitamin C is an ideal supplement for people whose busy lifestyles lead to irregular eating habits, who miss meals, who are elderly and find preparing nourishing meals difficult, who are convalescing or who find it difficult to ensure a regular intake of vitamin C throughout the day. The recommended daily doses are:

- Vitamin C-Time 500 mg with bioflavonoids – one tablet every six hours
- Vitamin C-Time 1000 mg with bioflavonoids – one tablet every six hours (up to a maximum of three a day)
- Vitamin C-Time 1500 mg with bioflavonoids – one tablet every six hours (up to a maximum of two per day).

Vitamin B Complex

The B group of vitamins is a collection of essential nutrients that have certain characteristics in common. They are all non-protein, nitrogen-containing, water-soluble substances found in foods such as meats, soya, wholegrains, cereals, vegetables and brewer's yeast. The B complex functions in the body as a group of vitamins.

While chemically distinct from one another, the ways in which the B vitamins work in the body are closely related, the metabolisms of folic acid and vitamin B12, for example, being closely connected. Similarly, vitamins B2 and B3 are required for the activation of vitamin B6, and vitamin B3 can be manufactured from other dietary agents provided that there is adequate B6.

The effective production of energy from foodstuffs relies on the presence of many of the B vitamins. It is in this process that they act as co-enzymes for macronutrient breakdown or catabolism, releasing energy. The B vitamins also contribute to the health and maintenance of the adrenal glands, the liver, the skin and the hair, as well as to the effective production of red blood cells and haemoglobin. It is in the production of new cells that specific B vitamins have been highlighted as being of vital importance before and during pregnancy.

Members of the B vitamin group are also used to maintain the health of the nervous system. They are essential to enable the cells of the nervous system to take up oxygen. The primary and best remedy available in biological medicine for the treatment of painful inflammation of the nerves, as well as for strengthening the entire nervous system, is a steady supply of vitamin B. It is also a help to those who suffer from poor stomach and bowel action and the lack of appetite connected with these disorders. In cases of circulatory disorders and heart trouble, prescribed natural remedies will act faster and better if vitamin B is taken at the same time. In the past, explorers on Arctic and Himalayan expeditions took along supplies of yeast extract for the sake of its concentrated nutrients and its sufficient amount of vitamin B.

If not enough is present in the diet, a product containing the B complex vitamins may be chosen by anyone with a demanding lifestyle, those with endocrine imbalances, those with a poor dietary intake and heavy drinkers.

Lamberts offer two B complex products, both of which are yeast free:

- B-50 complex – recommended daily intake – one tablet
- B-100 complex – recommended daily intake – one tablet

The individual B vitamins are described below.

Vitamin B1

Vitamin B1, or thiamine, is considered to be the anti-beriberi vitamin. *Beri* is a Hindustani word referring to a sheep's fetlock, and in Sinhalese, *beri* means weakness. The weakness or loss of energy experienced by those whose diet is based on white rice leads to a partial paralysis of the limbs, making patients drag their feet in a similar way to the sheep. For this reason the disease, which is caused by a dietary deficiency of vitamin B1, has become known as beriberi. Vitamin B1 deficiency also shows up with cracked and bleeding gums and lips.

Vitamin B1 is a complex substance that takes part in the breaking down of carbon–carbon bonds and is a co-factor for the carbohydrate-splitting enzyme pyruvic decarboxylase. Vitamin B1 is thus used to release energy in cells, working in co-operation with other members of the vitamin B complex, particularly vitamin B2 (riboflavin) and vitamin B3 (niacin).

Vitamin B1 is contained in the aleurone layer of cereals, a good quantity also being present in yeast. Vitamin B1 may be deficient in those who smoke or drink heavily, and those whose work is particularly strenuous. If supplements are needed, the recommended daily intake is one 100 mg capsule.

Vitamin B2

Vitamin B2 (riboflavin) is one of an important family of compounds known as the flavins, which are involved in the electron transport mechanism of the respiratory chain and are therefore essential in releasing energy in cells. Most intestinal flora synthesise riboflavin, as do germinating seeds, and it is stored in both the liver and the heart. The recommended daily supplement is one or two 50 mg capsules.

Vitamin B3

Vitamin B3 (niacin) appears in several different forms, all of which can be referred to as niacin. One of the forms is nicotinamide, which is needed to break down amino acids from proteins, and to synthesise and degrade fatty acids. Nicotinamide supplementation is recommended to be one or two 250 mg tablets daily.

Vitamin B5

We cannot synthesise this vitamin (pantothenic acid), but it is ubiquitous throughout the plant and animal kingdom. It is used in the production of corticosteroid hormones by the adrenal glands and in cholesterol metabolism. During demanding situations, this vitamin often enables us to cope better biochemically. The recommended daily supplement is one tablet of calcium pantothenate 500 mg.

Vitamin B6

Vitamin B6 is a family of three closely related compounds: pyridoxine, pyridoxal and pyridoxamine. Pyridoxine is involved in more bodily functions than any other single nutrient. Vitamin B6 helps with the transport of the commonly deficient mineral magnesium, and is necessary in the production of hydrochloric acid in the stomach, as well as in the absorption of fats and proteins. The synthesis of many protein-based substances such as hormones and neurotransmitters relies on the availability of vitamin B6 and zinc. Vitamin B6 is also concerned with the conversion of the amino acid tryptophan to vitamin B3. The recommended daily intake of vitamin B6 is one 50 mg tablet.

Pyridoxine itself is an alcohol, but its active form is either the corresponding aldehyde or the amine, and each must be in the form of a phosphate for optimum bio-availability. The active form of the vitamin is pyridoxal phosphate (P5P), however, other types of vitamin B6 being converted into this form in the cells of the body. P5P plays a major part in the metabolism of protein as a co-factor in transamination reactions necessary to change one amino acid to another in their synthesis. High-protein diets, therefore, demand a high P5P level and hence a high vitamin B6 intake. Pyridoxal-5-Phosphate Plus supplementation of one or two capsules a day can be taken.

Vitamin B12

Vitamin B12 (cyanocobalamin) is a complex substance, first isolated in 1948 from liver, which contains the mineral cobalt at its centre. It is needed for the synthesis of DNA and for normal metabolism in nerve tissue. Vitamin B12 principally participates in the rapid regeneration of bone marrow and red blood cells.

A doctor friend told me that a certain patient's anaemic condition had its root in a vegetarian diet. This patient, who was otherwise quite healthy, was unable to overcome the anaemia, and the doctor was adamant that the man should add meat to his diet because it is rich in haematinic vitamin B12. But when the doctor found out that I'd been a vegetarian since I was seventeen, and had a constant healthy haemoglobin count and otherwise excellent blood, he was astonished and had to change his opinion.

A healthy vegetarian diet must include plenty of green vegetables and culinary herbs, such as cress and parsley, because these contain sufficiently high levels of vitamin B12. All these green herbs, in particular parsley, stimulate the kidneys and urination, and should therefore be used regularly rather than as just an occasional garnish on prepared dishes. In fact, your health will benefit greatly if you chop up some kitchen herbs daily, mixing them in your salads and cottage cheese and sprinkling them over vegetable and potato dishes. You can ensure a regular intake of these green herbs by using the herbal seasoning salt Herbamare, which is made from fresh green herbs. If you use natural products regularly in your kitchen you will reduce the risk of succumbing to vitamin deficiency. If a supplement is needed of vitamin B12, 100 μg, one tablet a day, is recommended.

Folic acid

Folic acid is formed from glutamic acid, para-aminobenzoic acid and another group of organic substances. It is synthesised by intestinal bacteria and is involved in cell division in both plants and animals. The metabolism of folic acid is closely linked to that of vitamin B12. Folic acid, choline, lecithin and biotin (described below) tend to be found in the same foodstuffs as the B vitamins. The recommended supplement of folic acid is one 400 µg tablet daily.

Choline and inositol

Choline is a much-discussed, vitamin-like substance. It is a natural component of lecithin, which participates in fat metabolism, particularly in relation to the liver. This activity of choline is shared with inositol. It is the precursor of acetylcholine, an important neurotransmitter. The recommended daily intake of choline 250 mg/ inositol 250 mg is one tablet daily.

Lecithin

Lecithin, technically called a phospholipid, is one of the richest natural sources of phosphatidyl choline and inositol. Both nutrients play an important role in the healthy functioning of the nervous system and gastrointestinal tract.

Use one or two tablespoons of soya lecithin granules daily, sprinkled onto cereals, stirred into fruit juices or added as a thickener to soups and casseroles.

Biotin

Biotin is produced by intestinal bacteria, antibiotics and other medication often affecting its production. The co-enzyme properties of biotin enable it to metabolise carbohydrate and protein for energy release and to take part in the production of prostaglandins – hormone-like substances – from essential fatty acids. In the body, it is primarily used to assist with the normal growth and development of the skin, hair, nerves and bone marrow. One to three capsules of biotin 500 µg are recommended daily.

Vitamin D

'Vitamin D' actually refers to a group of closely related substances involved in the metabolism of calcium and phosphorus in the body (increasing their uptake and decreasing their excretion) and therefore in the formation of healthy bones.

It might seem as if this would be more important in children than in those over fifty, but, as I discuss at more length in the chapter on osteoporosis, maintaining the quality of bone is of vital importance as we get older, especially for women, who are especially vulnerable about the time of the menopause.

Sunlight plays a part by activating a vitamin D precursor in the skin, but rather than heading for Spain in the winter and running the risk of skin cancer, we can boost our vitamin D intake by eating the right foods, and by supplements if necessary. Oily fish such as mackerel, herring and kipper are high in vitamin D, as are salmon, fish-liver oils and egg yolks.

Having looked at vitamins, we will now move onto minerals and trace elements, also vital in sufficient quantities for good health. Again, these may become deficient because of stress, chemical pollutants, processed foods and so on. They can be found naturally in a wide range of foods.

Minerals, which cannot be synthesised by the human body, are essential factors in human nutrition – certainly every bit as important as vitamins. Minerals are natural components of the chemical catalysts (enzymes) that regulate physiological functions. They are used in the upkeep of the central nervous system, the growth, maintenance and repair of tissues, and hormone production.

A trace element is a mineral for which the human daily requirement is less than 25 mg.

Potassium

This product may take part in the body's water balance regulatory system, in maintaining a normal heart rate and in keeping muscle function healthy. Supplements may be appropriate for people using diuretics (excepting potassium-sparing diuretics) or those losing a lot of fluid through physical activity. It is very important for bones too, so supplementation is beneficial in those suffering with arthritic or rheumatic conditions. As it cannot exist as a mineral–amino acid combination, potassium is available in citrated form, the recommended daily intake being one or two tablets of 200 mg potassium citrate daily.

GTF chromium

Glucose tolerance factor (GTF) includes vitamin B3 an a trio of amino acids in its molecule; it is often referred to as a polynicotinate. Chromium is known to take part in enabling the cells to take up glucose for energy release, and is also believed to be involved in the synthesis of fatty acids and cholesterol, taking part in the activity of insulin. Other similar compounds, such as picolinates, may be fairly well absorbed, but research shows they have little or no effect on insulin activity. The recommended daily intake of GTF chromium is one 200 μg capsule daily.

Iodine (kelp extract)

The seaweed kelp acts as a collecting organism, extracting components from seawater and concentrating them. One of the most important constituents of kelp is iodine, which is required by the thyroid gland for the production of thyroxine. This hormone increases the body's general metabolism, improves blood flow and enhances the breakdown of food. It has also been shown to reduce cholesterol levels, and helps to support the activity of the endocrine glands, which will be of benefit to any woman going through the menopause.

Kelp is often chosen by:

- anyone wanting a natural source supplement
- those who eat little or no fish, cereals, fruit and vegetables

- slimmers and those dieting to maintain a stable weight, to ensure an adequate intake of iodine
- people wishing to maintain the health of their scalp and hair
- teenagers and young people who have a finicky diet (especially during growing periods – important to know for their parents!)

Lamberts iodine tablets contain kelp in the form of dried *Ascophyllum nodosum* and dry extract of *Fucus vesiculosis*, and are carefully prepared to ensure that 150 μg of iodine are provided in every tablet. One to three tablets are recommended daily.

Manganese

Manganese can contribute towards the raw materials essential for the making and functioning of many enzymes in the body, including those involved in the synthesis of cartilage components as well as one of the superoxide dismutases; these help to prevent the formation of a cascade of free radicals, which can cause tissue damage when present in excess. Manganese 5 mg (as an amino acid chelate) is supplemented as one to three capsules daily.

Zinc

The principal role of any trace element is that of promoting the catalytic action of enzymes. Zinc is an invaluable mineral taking part in dehydrogenation and peptidase processes, being specific for the enzyme that removes the terminal amino acid from one particular end of a peptide. It is also specific for the enzyme that is responsible for the ultimate elimination of carbon dioxide from an organism, and for the production of hydrochloric acid in the parietal cells of the stomach. Zinc is an integral part of insulin, the main hormone in the body involved in glucose metabolism and used in the treatment of diabetes. In addition, zinc is essential for all protein synthesising the body.

Zinc is thus involved in:

- maintaining the gastrointestinal wall
- the health of the prostate gland

- protein synthesis and collagen formation
- a healthy skin
- the maintenance of a healthy immune system
- tissue repair
- taste and smell
- the maintenance of a proper concentration of vitamin A in the blood

Any extra physical or mental demands made on the body can increase the need for zinc or cause our bodies to lose extra zinc, whereas phytate- and fibre-rich foods, such as chapattis, and fruit and vegetables respectively, inhibit the absorption of zinc from food.

Zinc supplements are given as citrate, this part appearing to help in the absorption of zinc through the gut wall. Zinc citrate appears to be highly bio-available, the recommended daily intake being:

- zinc citrate 50 mg – one capsule
- zinc citrate 15 mg – one capsule

Magnesium

Magnesium is the second most abundant mineral inside cells. It is needed for the release of calcitonin, the hormone that encourages calcium to be deposited in the bones rather than in the soft tissues of the body, and is therefore essential for bone growth. By activating the enzymes that are necessary for the breakdown of carbohydrates, magnesium also plays an important role in energy metabolism. It is a vital enzyme co-factor in the manufacture of specific proteins from DNA, the nucleic acid code that governs the growth of all cells.

Magnesium also exerts its action through the proper functioning of nerves and muscles, especially those of the heart, as, unless there is sufficient magnesium, a stimulated nerve cannot return to its resting state.

Magnesium is therefore essential for:

- bone growth and health
- the metabolism of carbohydrate to release energy

- nerve impulse transmission and brain function
- normal muscle function, including that of the heart

Magnesium intake in the diet has declined sharply during the last few decades in developed countries as a result of declining energy expenditure and the refining and processing of food, which often removes the mineral-rich parts of the food.

Lamberts amino acid chelate, containing 150 mg of magnesium, is a highly effective formulation when a supplement is needed. Many experts believe that an amino acid chelate offers the most absorbable form of magnesium, as this compound mimics the magnesium that occurs in food. This product combines high technical advantage with excellent value for money, making it the first choice for many nutritionists selecting a magnesium product. Since magnesium is needed for steady brain functioning, many people choose to take magnesium supplements before they go to bed at night in order that can work to its best uninterrupted. The recommended daily intake is one or two tablets.

Calcium and magnesium combinations

Calcium is the most abundant mineral in the body, with 99 per cent being present in the bones and teeth. The other 1 per cent plays a vital role in the transmission of nerve impulses to the muscles of the body and heart. Calcium and magnesium are often linked together, probably because of their combined roles in ensuring bone health.

Calcium & Magnesium ACC is a product that provides calcium and magnesium as amino acid chelates in a ratio of 2:1. Calcium amino acid chelate is the nearest supplement to milk calcium. The recommended daily intake is from two to six tablets.

Mineral complexes

In my clinics, my personal preference is to use mineral and trace element complexes such as Lamberts Health Insurance Plus, available from some chemists or from the manufacturer. Lamberts also offer two mineral complexes – Mega Mineral Complex and Trace Mineral Complex – differing mainly in the amount of calcium and magnesium provided. Both products have trace minerals at relevant levels.

Mega Mineral Complex is probably one of the most comprehensive high-potency mineral formulae available. It can be used when the vitamins in a supplement regime are supplied separately, and, if it is combined with one of Lamberts high-potency vitamin formulae, such as Multi-Max, a comprehensive potent supplement regime can be created. The recommended daily intake is two tablets.

Lamberts Trace Mineral Complex supplies all the most important trace minerals along with useful amounts of calcium and magnesium. One tablet daily is the recommended intake.

Lamberts Health Insurance Plus, as the name suggests, contains a broad spectrum of nutrients, all presented at sensible but relevant levels. This formula will help to safeguard against deficiencies in the diet. Rich in protective anti-oxidant nutrients, this formula also boasts a good mineral mix, the minerals being presented in compounds known to be well absorbed, such as chelates and gluconates. Since the change to amino acid chelate (ACC) form of magnesium, Health Insurance Plus has become unbeatable in terms of the quality of mineral compounds used: magnesium is rarely present in every multiple formula at both a useful level and in a proven absorbable form. Health Insurance Plus is also presented in a hypoallergenic preparation.

This product is suitable as a nutritional safeguard for persons with inadequate diets, immune dysfunction, chronic illnesses and periods of rapid growth, as well as for the elderly. One or two tablets are recommended daily.

Another mineral complex is Imuno-Strength, a special preparation containing vitamins, minerals and herbal extracts that I have formulated myself for Nature's Best, as it is important for people to be able to provide a tremendous boost to their immune system when necessary. The immune system is a multi-faceted, highly sophisticated system that helps to protect our bodies and keep them healthy. The maintenance of an efficient immune system, dependent upon adequate intakes of certain vitamins and minerals that are included in Imuno-Strength, is vital. The recommended daily intake is two tablets.

Doctor's Choice for Women is a daily multiple formula designed specifically for women by Dr Michael T. Murray that can be obtained from many chemists and health food shops. It is a gender-specific supplement – one to three tablets daily – that provides extra calcium and iron, and a full range of B vitamins. It provides a real boost for women, especially when their immune system is functioning poorly, and gives wonderful results.

Today, we are certainly more interested in our health than ever before, but it must be remembered that good health cannot be achieved just by taking vitamin, mineral and trace element supplements – a good underlying diet is essential. Although it is not always easy to put this into practice, our aim must be to obtain as many of these nutrients as possible naturally, before considering taking supplements. With this basis of a healthy diet, you will be equipped to enter this new, exciting phase of your life.

6

How do I look after my weight?

Weight concern is a subject that touches most people. Our affluent Western society makes it possible to overeat – and many of us do just that! Until recently, women's magazines often published tables telling us what we should weigh depending on whether we had a heavy, medium or light bone structure. These weights were, however, so low that they were difficult to attain and almost impossible to sustain.

Nowadays, there is an acceptable range of body weight, which is measured by the body mass index (BMI). To find out your BMI, take the square of your height in metres and divide it into your body weight in kilogrammes. For example, if you measure 1.67 m and your weight is 62 kg, your BMI is:

$$\frac{62}{1.67 \times 1.67} = 22.2$$

$$\therefore \text{ BMI} = 22$$

Your BMI must lie in the range 20 to 25 in order to ensure that you are the correct weight. If it is less, you are underweight and must do something about it as being too light is as dangerous as being too heavy. If your BMI is above 25, you are either overweight or obese, depending on how much over your desired weight you are.

It is unfortunate that 'overweight' and 'obese' are often used without thought as they are not synonymous. 'Obesity' reflects a definite clinical situation in which men have a body fat in excess of 20 per cent of their total weight while women require a body fat excess of 30 per cent to be classified as obese. If you fall into the overweight category, your body fat is above the desirable level, but this is not associated with the same degree of medical complications as associated with clinical obesity.

If you are underweight, for example after an illness or operation, or with a chronic condition such as emphysema or depression, you will need to increase the amount of food you eat if you want to gain weight, always remembering the principles for healthy eating that we outlined in the previous two chapters. Loss of appetite can be helped by twice a day taking one 15 mg capsule of zinc along with fifteen drops of the herbal remedy centaurium. This helps to increase the secretion of digestive enzymes and quicken gut motility, thus improving the breakdown of food.

Unfortunately, however, as weight tends to increase with age anyway, many of us have the opposite problem, so in this chapter we will concentrate on keeping the weight down to the healthy range, so that we can look and feel our best.

Start by taking stock of yourself in a full-length mirror. All right, you hair may be a mess, your skin is a disaster area, your clothes don't hang properly and you feel far from 100 per cent! But these are the negative aspects; this is only what you are starting with. Remember that whether it is one stone or six stones that you have to lose, it doesn't matter. One person's single stone is just as depressing to him or her as someone else's six; the feeling is just the same.

So take another look in the mirror and think positively. You may have beautiful teeth or hands and not everyone with a weight problem has pasty skin and lank hair. Stand straight with your shoulders down and the crown of your head reaching for the ceiling, your 'tail' and tummy tucked in, and your knees unlocked. Note how much better your clothes look.

While you are working on your new figure and waiting for it to appear (which takes patience), concentrate on grooming. We all know people who are much too fat or much too thin yet look fabulous. Think of them and, as a temporary measure, try to imitate them. You will feel much better about yourself for having done something positive and put yourself in a much better position for the new life ahead of you.

So you want to get fit and lose weight – don't think that it will be easy. You will have to learn about your body and what makes it tick if the new you is to be a permanent fixture. Dieting, diet foods, fitness centres and diet pills are big business. If you believe all you read about these diet aids, you might think that obesity and weight problems should be a thing of the past, but obesity is a big problem that is getting bigger.

According to the University of Sheffield's own publication, *Focus on Medicine*, the prevalence of obesity in the UK is increasing at an alarming rate. Researchers at the Centre for Human Nutrition are investigating the mechanisms by which people of normal weight regulate their calorie intake. It is hoped that, by understanding these processes, it will be possible to gain information concerning the cause of obesity. Another team at the same centre is looking into the gut's behavioral responses to food and how it adapts to special nutritional conditions, such as an overconsumption of fat.

It appears to be a standard joke that if your doctor is in doubt, he or she blames a virus, but joking apart, there is mounting evidence that a virus known as AD-36, which is responsible for obesity in some animals, could be present in the bodies of obese subjects. The report published in the medical journal *The Lancet* showed that an analysis of 199 blood samples from obese volunteers proved positive for the Ad-36 virus in 15 per cent of those tested whereas none of the 45 'lean' volunteers had the virus. The researchers suggested that this new finding could help to explain the rapid worldwide increase in the condition over the past ten years.

Recent research has also thrown new light onto the issue of eating disorders, which often show up by a change in weight. These disorders often develop from an unhealthy attitude to food triggered by an unconscious mental disorder. Sometimes, it is simply boredom, but more frequently it is something deeper, such as a feeling of inadequacy or rejection. In cases of bulimia and anorexia nervosa, body image can be the problem. Recognising and correcting the root of the disorder goes a long way to curing it. Initial success in treatment is encouraging, and since success breeds success, this can trigger the right frame of mind, enabling the person with the affliction to lose or gain the necessary weight. An optimistic attitude goes a long way in bringing about a cure. Sometimes the reason for the disorder is deep-seated and counselling is necessary.

Is there, though, a healthy fatness and an unhealthy fatness? For years, people have argued about their shape, size and level of health. Some people appear to be overweight but live a long and apparently healthy life, free from the complications associated with being fat, while others fall prey to their bodily excess in their early years. This obviously raises the question of whether there is or can be a 'healthy' fat frame.

Dr David Ashton from Imperial College School of Medicine in London has shed some light on this dilemma. He explains that there are basically two types of fat person, those with android (central) obesity and those with gynoid (peripheral) obesity. The typical android person has a protruding belly – the classic beer belly – while those in the gynoid group carry their weight more on their hips. These people do not have a high risk of heart disease, while their android counterparts need to be aware that they are at a higher risk of elevated cholesterol level, diabetes and raised blood pressure as well as other risk factors associated with coronary heart disease. So your health may in part depend on where your weight tends to accumulate.

In addition, men and women are very different in their response to weight control; they cannot and will not lose weight at the same rate. This has nothing to do with the willpower to succeed: it is basic physiology. Men have a different body composition, with a greater lean muscle mass (in the region of 20–35 per cent more than women), as well as different hormonal (especially testosterone) and metabolic influences that control the body's desire to maintain a certain amount of body fat. Women have an additional problem in that they tend to put on extra weight around the time of the menopause as their hormone balance changes.

The most metabolically active tissues are the lean (muscle) tissues. The amount of lean tissue determines the metabolic rate, that is, the calorie-burning capacity of the body. The greater amount of lean muscle, the more energy (calories) we burn even at rest, the body's metabolic 'tick-over' rate being increased. By virtue of their greater muscle mass and higher testosterone level, most men have a biological advantage over women when it comes to weight control and performance in weight loss programmes – the difference between men and woman really is more than skin deep.

Just mention the word 'dieting' and people run for their calorie counters, totting up their daily intake as they go. Men generally consume 500–1000 more calories per day than women. When a man reduces his calorie intake by 1000 calories, he is still left eating about 2000–2500 calories worth of food daily. On the other hand, when a woman cuts her intake by the same 1000 calories, she really feels the difference – there is hardly anything that she can eat without spoiling her diet. This is a serious problem and can lead to true nutritional deficiencies, which in turn hinder the weight loss process.

By following male dieters, women can easily suffer from 'starvation syndrome' characterised by a lowering of the metabolic rate. The body is a master of nutritional survival! When food is scarce, it is senseless to keep the metabolic fires raging as this only burns up the precious stored energy that is keeping the body insulated from the cold or heat. Lowering the metabolic rate thus lowers the calorific needs of the body, a necessary survival step during starvation. It appears to be a biological characteristic that the female metabolic system is particularly sensitive to developing 'starvation syndrome' and its metabolic consequences.

There has been a suggestion that repeated crash diets can 'scar' the metabolic system in such a way that it becomes oversensitive to changes in food intake (and therefore energy intake), making the classic roller-coaster gains and losses experienced by long-term dieters a real problem as the metabolic systems 'thermostat' becomes reset by 'crash' dieting. The low calorie intake means that the metabolic rate falls and muscle is lost. As more muscle is lost, the metabolic rate falls still further, so when you eat more, the calories cannot be burnt off, and you will gain weight again.

So the key to getting the metabolism to work in our favour is to get it to burn the food calories more efficiently. This cannot, however, be done quickly and is definitely not achieved by taking diet pills. The only way to achieve it is by observing a slow and balanced weight loss programme, coming to terms with the fact that a healthy weight loss is a slow weight loss. Exercise, too, is involved as it will increase our metabolic rate. And remember this approach is not a temporary measure but a new way of life.

So let's look at what we can actually *do* to help to control our weight. The obvious area to tackle is diet, as if we take more calories in than we use, we will naturally put on weight; it must, however, be remembered that someone who is more physically active will need more calories.

Getting the proportion of protein and carbohydrates correct is one of the keys to a successful diet. Over the past five years, diet trends have swung towards a high complex carbohydrate diet (that is, one including foods high in starch, such as pasta, pulses and so on). As with all things in life, though, too much of a good thing can end up being bad! Carbohydrates are great for energy, providing four calories per gram, but as good as they are, we need to keep them in balance with other nutrients.

Protein, for example, is essential for health and also provides four calories of energy per gram, but using protein for energy is not the best use of raw materials, nor is this the prime function of protein. In addition to its vital contribution to growth and repair, protein is essential for water balance, which is one of the reasons why carbohydrates and proteins should be eaten together in a balanced amount. For every 0.5–1 kg (1 lb) of carbohydrate stored in the body, a further 1.5 kg (3 lb) of water is retained. Protein is, therefore, necessary to help regulate excessive water retention. The balance of carbohydrate and protein is also important in the regulation of the blood sugar level. If this swings up and down, so do our moods, emotions and eating habits.

Having said all this, the question remains, 'What should we eat?' In the past, a diet consisting of about 1000 calories per day was recommended in order to lose weight. It was stressed that those thousand calories had to be properly balanced so that they contained proteins, fats and carbohydrates. This, of course, worked but was very boring and one had to be very determined in order to succeed. In addition to this sensible diet, all sorts of fad diets have arisen, for example the diet that suggested eating one food and one food only

– sometimes even chocolate – for a whole day. Although any diet that is not properly balanced will cause a weight loss, it will not leave us feeling and looking healthy.

So first, think about your lifestyle. It doesn't matter whether you are a nibbler or a three-meals-a-day person, as long as there is order in your life. Nothing works better than routine. I have heard some people say, 'If I only had myself to cater for, it would be much easier,' and others say, 'If only I had somebody to cook for, it would be much better.' Whatever your circumstances, not being organised will hold you back.

The latest research shows that in order to live a healthy life, we should refrain from sugar and saturated fats. If we follow this advice, we will feel better but will not necessarily lose or gain weight, so we have to use additional methods. Although we need to eat a little less than we have been doing, there are some foods that can be eaten in any amount without doing any harm. Vegetables, used with low-fat dressings or made into soup, are excellent fillers. Fruit is a good substitute for biscuits and cakes, but remember that because of its sugar content, fruit can also add weight if too much is eaten. Potatoes are not the evil-doers that they were once thought to be, nor are baked beans. A lunch consisting of a baked potato filled with cottage cheese or baked beans, with a side salad and followed by a piece of fruit, is a healthy meal that should see you through the afternoon. It is advisable to avoid pork, bacon and gammon; although these are not always fatty, they are high in animal acids and slow down weight loss.

If you eat fresh foods, you will find that you are more easily satisfied; any wholesome food freshly cooked is good. Use vegetable cooking oil or olive oil sparingly, and avoid adding sugar. You will soon find that food cooked in this manner tastes much better. Learn to use herbs and spices. Using a wok will make quick meals tastier, and the crispiness of the vegetables makes them a lot more attractive. A few adjustments to our daily food intake can make a big difference to our weight, almost without our noticing. Use skimmed milk instead of full or semi-skimmed milk. Light margarine is a good substitute for the full-fat version that you may have been using. Low-fat salad dressings and yoghurt help, too.

Although I am not a promoter of artificial sweeteners, they are better than sugar. However, if you are fighting a sugar addiction, it is better to use unsweetened food rather than keep the taste for sugar alive by using artificial sweeteners. Try it for yourself. Low fat and natural yoghurt with fresh fruit tastes much better than the low-fat and low-calorie varieties on the supermarket shelves.

It is a good idea to read ingredient labels on all that you buy. If there is too much sugar or saturated fat, forget it – shop around for a healthier variety.

The most difficult aspect of reforming your life is tackling your addictions. This is mostly an addiction to sugar or fizzy drinks. Remember – and this is the good news – that an addiction takes only about two or three weeks to break. If you can stop eating or drinking your favourite vice for a few weeks, the desire for it will leave you. If your addiction is fizzy drinks, do not switch to low-calorie substitutes. All fizzy drinks contain a high level of phosphates, so whichever you drink is bad for you.

When you are trying to break your addiction the almost irresistible desire to indulge with unexpectedly hit you now and again. Be ready to occupy yourself by calling a friend, doing some craftwork, or weeding the garden. Believe me, when you get as far as doing something, the desire will pass.

There are, of course, many people who prefer to follow a regular eating pattern and feel that the stick behind the door is necessary in keeping them strictly to a diet. Many years ago, we formulated a very successful diet: by adhering to this you will notice significant results very quickly. The secret of the diet is to follow the guidelines regarding daily and weekly allowances very carefully. This can be combined with acupressure to stimulate the points in the ear that improve the metabolism and quell the appetite. Botanical Slimming Formula (available from chemists and health food stores), containing several herbal ingredients to cleanse the body, improve the metabolism and help to absorb and burn up fat, can be taken at the same time.

This diet is presented as the Jan De Vries Healthy Eating Plan. Remember that success with this diet, as with all diets, can only be achieved by carefully weighing your food each time. All soups must be made using stock cubes and vegetables only, and cream soups may be made using part of your daily milk allowance.

The daily allowances, which must be consumed within a period of twenty-four hours, are:

- milk – ½ pint of fresh, or ¾ pint of semi-skimmed, or 1 pint skimmed milk, or two cartons of plain or low-fat fruit yoghurt
- wholemeal bread – 3 weighed ounces, *not* slices
- meat – 4 oz, or 6 oz of fish, or 4 oz of smoked fish, or 5 oz of chicken
- fruit – three portions

Weekly allowances, which must be consumed within one week, are:

- butter or margarine – 4 oz, or 8 oz of 'Gold'
- cheese – 8 oz
- eggs (optional) – up to seven

The following can be exchanged for 1 oz of bread:

- potato – 3 oz
- two crispbread or crackers or water biscuits or two plain biscuits
- breakfast cereal – 1 oz of any sort except sugar coated
- porridge – 1 oz uncooked weight
- cooked rice – two dessertspoonfuls

Vegetarian substitutes for animal protein can be accounted for in this programme to provide an adequate amount of protein in your day-to-day diet. The following foods are sources of protein:

- dairy foods – milk, cheese, yoghurt, fromage frais and eggs
- vegetable sources – lentils, nuts, grains, peas and beans
- soya, tofu and quorn

Eight ounces of the following cheeses is allowed:

- Caerphilly
- Camembert
- Cheshire
- cottage (4 oz only)
- Danish Blue
- Edam

- Gruyère
- Leicester
- Parmesan
- Roquefort
- Stilton
- Wensleydale
- smoked Austrian

There are no restrictions on most vegetables. Try:

- artichokes
- asparagus
- aubergines
- beansprouts
- beetroot
- broccoli
- brussel sprouts
- cabbage (any type)
- carrots
- cauliflower
- celery
- chicory
- courgettes
- cress
- cucumber
- leeks
- lettuce
- marrow
- mushrooms
- onions
- parsley
- parsnip
- peppers
- pickles
- pimentos
- radish
- runner beans
- spinach
- spring onions

- swede
- tomatoes

Avocado, baked beans (3–5 oz), broad, butter and haricot beans, chickpeas, peas and sweetcorn should be eaten in moderation.

Three portions of fruit should be eaten daily. A portion is:

- apple – one average
- apricots – two fresh
- bananas – one small
- blackberries – 4 oz
- cherries – 4 oz
- cooking apples – one large
- damsons – ten
- dates – 1 oz
- gooseberries – ten
- grapefruit – half
- grapes – 3 oz
- melon – one average slice
- orange – one average
- pineapple – one slice fresh
- plums – two fresh
- raisins – 1 oz
- raspberries – 5 oz
- rhubarb – 5 oz
- strawberries – 5 oz
- sultanas – 1 oz
- tangerines, etc. – two
- unsweetened juice – 110 ml (4 fl oz)

These drinks can be incorporated into your diet:

- Bovril
- coffee
- Energen 1 cal
- herb tea
- lemon juice
- low-calorie tonic water – although it is best to avoid fizzy drinks altogether

- Marmite
- Oxo
- Russian tea
- slimline drinks
- soda water
- tea
- tomato juice
- water

Salt, pepper, vinegar, mustard, lemon juice, herbs, spices and Worcestershire sauce can be used for seasoning.

You may eat as often as you like within your allowance time, but you must not eat fewer than three meals a day. If a food does not appear on the list, it should not be eaten without prior consultation.

Do not isolate yourself in following your new lifestyle: there is much more in the world that just food. If you are dining out, enjoy yourself. Enjoy the ambience of your surroundings, the company, the colours, the smells and the good conversation. And remember, always make yourself look attractive before you go out.

There is, however, not much point in trying to keep the weight off by dietary measures if you are not going to turn up the metabolic thermostat by increasing the lean tissue mass – yes, I mean take some regular exercise. Exercise is also conducive to positive thinking, which helps to make controlling your weight a bit more bearable.

It may take some willpower to persuade oneself into action as when too much weight is being carried, it is not easy to drag it around while exercising. So start with something simple but which you know you will achieve. Walking comes to mind. Begin gently and don't spend more than twenty minutes at a time on it. See how far you can walk in that time – ten minutes there, ten minutes back. Try to walk a little further each day within the same time limit. It is surprising how quickly you will find yourself stronger and lighter on your feet.

Swimming is also a good starting point because the water will support your weight, and you will be exercising all your muscles. The chapter on exercise will give you some more ideas and some recommendations on how much to exercise.

If you choose to join, for example, a keep-fit class, make sure that you join one suitable for your measure of fitness. Sometimes people feel self-conscious about joining classes when they are overweight, but you will be surprised to discover how many people in your class have the same problem.

Should you feel unsure about being able to exercise, consult your doctor and he or she will be able to advise you on what is best. It is good to think not so much about going on a diet in order to lose or gain weight but about a new beginning and a new you.

The metabolic thermostat can also be turned up by stimulating the thyroid. The chapter on exercise describes how sea-bathing can help here; alternatively, take four kelp tablets first thing in the morning with a cup of hot water.

Finally, we can summarise some important weight loss 'secrets':

- Drink plenty of water: about 1–1.5 litres (about 1½–2½ pints) of water daily. Don't confuse hunger with thirst.
- Don't cut your calorie intake to below 1000 per day as this will damage your metabolic rate and hinder your weight loss.
- Take regular exercise as this will boost your metabolism and help you to form more lean tissue, which further increases your metabolic rate.
- Don't weigh yourself daily. A healthy weight loss is a slow one as fat comes off very slowly.
- Try to eat a healthy diet that you can live with. Don't think of it as a diet just for weight loss, but use it as a way of life.
- Don't exclude fat totally from your diet. Instead, reduce it to about 15 per cent of your daily calorie intake and make it 'healthy' fat, best taken in the monounsaturated form such as olive oil.
- Keep well clear of sugar and so-called 'diet' foods and drinks.
- Include ample protein. This is needed for muscle formation, especially during an exercise programme.
- Increase your fibre intake, best taken from fruit and vegetables.
- Select an attainable weight and fitness goal and stick to your programme – you *will* succeed.

And when you succeed, you will notice the benefits in terms of how good you look and feel. In the next chapter, we will look at exercise, as we have said a vital part of any weight-control programme.

7

How do I exercise?

I have frequently observed older people who, despite their age, have still been able to exercise and are indeed as fit now as they were twenty years ago. In fact, I recall a lady I knew many years ago who was nearly ninety yet maintained a regular programme of exercise including yoga, walking and also some neck and back exercises, all of which helped to keep her going. Exercise exerts a powerful influence on our state of health, especially after the age of fifty, when it is highly necessary to exercise daily in order to keep fit and healthy.

Today, fitness is largely considered an integral part of our lives. Indeed, it has become big business as many people pursue the ideal of a fit and healthy body. The vascular system, the lymphatic system, the circulatory system, the digestive system, the immune system and the respiratory system are all profoundly dependent upon physical activity for their efficient functioning. On an emotional level, we benefit immensely from the reduction of stress and anxiety, lethargy and depression that exercise brings. It can also provide significant relief to those suffering from insomnia and irritability.

Different types of exercise all have their own particular benefits. The amount of oxygen generated during yoga, for example, is very important for the circulation. In addition, the hormonal system also benefits. During the menopause, when there is a decrease in the levels of female hormones secreted by the ovaries, the body's muscle tone, especially in the pelvic area, degenerates. This can often be helped by walking, swimming, cycling and tennis, as these – aerobic – sports encourage the blood flow of nutrients to the pelvic area and therefore help to maintain the health of the tissues. Aerobic exercises are those increasing the heart rate and pulse for at least twenty minutes. They are important to keep the heart fit and healthy.

As Gloria writes, we do not need to think about pumping iron three times a week in a gym, but about simple exercise that we can introduce to our lives. Probably the most effective is walking, so the more you walk to the shops or with the dog, the better. Walking is a load-bearing exercise which is wonderful for keeping the bones as dense and strong as possible. It is good news indeed that everyday activities such as walking, gardening and climbing stairs can help to tone up your cardiovascular system. In fact, any activity that leaves you feeling warm and slightly out of breath is good for you. If you exercise moderately for thirty minutes at least three times a week, you can almost halve your risk of a heart attack compared with someone who is physically inactive. The trick is to choose something with which you feel comfortable and which you enjoy doing regularly.

Health problems such as osteoporosis, overweight and heart disease can all be improved by regular walking, cycling, tennis, dancing or golfing. T'ai chi, yoga or other disciplined forms of exercise are also ideal. Swimming is excellent as the water supports your weight, thus protecting your bones and joints. You will also be exercising all your muscles.

Another form of light aerobic exercise is dancing, line-dancing being one type that is also great fun. This is done to country and western music and has the advantage of being enjoyed in a group. Unlike heavy aerobic exercise, it is possible to line-dance for hours and still feel good. Joining a keep-fit class also makes exercising fun, but make sure that you join a class that is suitable for your level of fitness. Your doctor can give you advice on what might be best for you.

Flexibility in the joints can be improved by carrying out simple movements. For example, the ankles, knees and toes can be exercised by walking on your toes or wiggling them as if you are playing the piano. Try rotating the ankles twenty times in each direction to loosen them up.

Abdominal exercises – done by breathing in through the nose deep into the stomach, and then out through the mouth – are necessary for good muscular control and help to protect the back.

There is no excuse for avoiding a regular work out, even if you stay at home. As Gloria said above, you no longer have to 'go for the burn' – that approach fizzled out long ago. Current thinking is that we need instead to take regular aerobic-style exercise; the Health Education Authority recommends about 20 minutes of aerobic-style exercise undertaken three times a week. To be efficient, you will need to raise your heart rate to about 60–70 per cent of your maximal heart rate (MHR). MHR is the number of times your heart can pump in one minute, and can be estimated simply by subtracting your age in years from 220. Once you have determined this figure, you can establish a target heart rate (THR). In a fifty-two year old subject for example:

MHR = 220–52 = 168 beats per minute

THR, taken as 60 per cent of MHR = 101 beats per minute

THR, taken at 70 per cent of MHR = 118 beats per minute

As your level of fitness increases, so does the length of exercise time before you reach your THR.

As a rule of thumb, low-intensity, long-duration exercise maximises the burning of stored body fat, which is important if you are also trying to lose weight. As the exercise level increases to about 80–85% of your MHR, the emphasis shifts towards the aerobic style of fitness and cardiovascular training. Workouts at this level are definitely *not* recommended for beginners. To maximise weight loss, it is recommended that you exercise at least four times a week for about half an hour, but be sure to stay within your THR.

One of the most efficient forms of home exercise equipment is the skiing machine. Such equipment allows the exerciser to work all areas of the body while monitoring the pulse rate, which makes keeping within the safety limits as calculated by the THR as easy as looking at your watch!

As exercise will help to improve health, stamina and flexibility, it is good to walk even very short distances and do any exercise that you are capable of doing, even if you cannot yet manage the harder exercise mentioned above. While exercising, play some music – which will help to maintain a sense of inner harmony – and also wear comfortable clothing. Remember to warm up and stretch prior to exercising and then stretch again afterwards; most people don't do this and many therefore become injured. Rest for a few minutes after exercising and do not hurry back to normal life. Use the Hara breathing exercises, which I describe below to help you to relax. In addition, make sure that you do your exercises *every* day.

Remember Gloria's tips to make you take more exercise without really noticing:

- walk up stairs instead of taking the lift or escalator
- walk or cycle reasonable distances instead of always taking the car
- go for a walk during your lunch break instead of going to the shops
- take up a hobby like dancing, swimming, golf, tennis or cycling
- try to build in a little exercise at least three times a week
- if you have a dog, take it for more walks than usual – your dog will love you for it too!

Exercises taken around the time of the menopause can be very beneficial in helping to prevent or alleviate many of the symptoms associated with the menopause – hot flushes, night sweats, vaginal irritation, depression, osteoporosis and cardio-vascular problems. The chapter on coping with the menopause goes into the problems that may occur in more detail.

For women, an important area is that of pelvic floor exercises. The pelvic floor consists of a group of muscles that form a sling across the base of the pelvis and support everything inside the pelvic cavity including the uterus, the bladder and part of the bowel. These muscles are involved in helping to stop and start the flow of urine.

Pelvic floor exercises consist of contacting and squeezing this group of muscles on a regular basis.

One of the best series of exercises is that devised by Dr Arnold Kegel. These exercises can also be practised during sexual intercourse. Try the following. Draw up the vaginal muscles, hold them for two to three seconds, and then relax them. Repeat this five to ten times. Squeeze the vaginal muscles firmly, hold them for a few seconds and then relax them. Repeat this five to ten times as well.

Other exercises can be done to help strengthen the thighs and abdomen. Pelvic rocking or tilting is very effective, and exercises can even be done while washing the dishes, waiting for the bus or even as you sit through a boring meeting!

It is also advantageous to enjoy regular sexual activity as women who remain sexually active experience fewer signs of vaginal ageing than celibate women.

Deep breathing exercises are equally as important as physical exercise, and I often ask patients whether they have ever taken the time to pay close attention to their breathing. Life and breathing are synonymous; life is breath, and its absence is death. Without oxygen, our bodies cannot function at their best, which means that breathing exercises are very important indeed.

In which part of his or her body does a newborn baby breathe? You will find that there is little movement of the chest but a rhythmic rise and fall slightly below the navel. As the child grows older and forms its own personality, this breathing pattern will change, usually rising from the navel upwards. Tense people tend to breathe high up in the chest, as do those suffering from asthma. What we need to do is reverse this pattern and make sure we breathe from our abdomens.

When working in a hospital, I once met a young doctor who performed more operations than any of her colleagues yet still looked fresh and relaxed at the end of the day. She told me that her breathing technique was based on Hara breathing exercises, and to this day I am grateful that I have managed to take a short course in this method of correct breathing. The technique involves too many exercises to mention here, but I would like to tell you about just one, which I practise most days.

About four o'clock in the afternoon, the time of day that I was born, I sometimes begin to feel a little tired. This, by the way, is an experience that many people encounter as the time of their birth approaches. I lie on the floor when I feel tired and tell myself to relax completely. My eyes are closed, and I tell every part of my body, from my head to toes, to relax until I feel as if I am sinking deeper and deeper into the floor. Then I place my left hand about half an inch beneath my navel and place my right hand over it. At that point, a magnetic ring on the vital centre of man – Hare – is formed. The Chinese have an old saying that the navel is the gate to all happiness, and certainly, by doing this exercise, one feels very relaxed. Next I breathe in slowly through my nose, filling my stomach with air and keeping my rib cage still. This sounds easier than it is, and it actually takes a little time to master properly.

Concentrate your mind on your stomach and breathe in slowly. Once your stomach is filled with air, round your lips and slowly breathe out, pulling your stomach flat. This can be done as often as desired. The sensation after finishing this exercise is normally either one of complete relaxation and the desire for a nice sleep, or of refreshment and the desire to return to work. I must stress that it should be performed naturally, as a baby would do. It sometimes helps to imagine yourself walking in a beautiful garden where you discover the wonderful scent of roses, which you inhale slowly.

In a very old but very good book entitled *Forever Young, Forever Healthy*, by Indra Devi, there is a wonderful exercise that I have taught to many people. Begin breathing by slightly contracting your throat (this will partly close the epiglottis) and slowly inhale a breath, keeping your mouth shut. You will hear a little hissing sound coming from the back of the throat. This is an indication that you are doing the breathing correctly. Do not raise your chest while inhaling, but let your rib cage expand at the sides. Now slowly exhale with the same hissing sound while contracting the rib cage and slightly pulling in your stomach.

You have just taken one deep breath. Did you feel the pressure of the inhalation and exhalation at the back of your palate and throat? If so, fine. Sniffing in through the nostrils is wrong, and the slight hissing noise is your confirmation that you have got it right. If, however, your throat is contracted too much, this slight hissing turns into snort; this is also wrong as it will strain the throat.

Now repeat the deep breathing by taking only three more

inhalations and exhalations, no more that this on your first time. You can repeat the same thing later on during the day and then again in the evening, but remember not to take more than four deep breaths each time.

To establish the rhythm of your breathing, place your third and fourth fingers on your wrist and listen to the pulse beat – count 1,2,3,4, 1,2,3,4 – several times. Now put your hands on your knees and start your deep breathing exercise, mentally counting four pulse beats while inhaling the breath and four pulse beats while exhaling it. Be sure not to accentuate the count of beats with your breath; the breath should flow smoothly. When inhaling, concentrate on the intake of fresh air filled with oxygen. Visualise it entering your lungs, and if you have a weak spot in your body, direct it mentally to that area.

Over the first month of doing this exercise, keep counting four pulse beats while inhaling and four while exhaling. Do not add an extra beat until you can do it very easily and without any effort. It may take over a month before you are able to increase the length of time for your inhalation and exhalation, but go slowly for maximum benefit.

As well as limiting the number of pulse beats you follow, for the first week, take only four breaths in one session. The second week, you can take five deep breaths. Continue adding one extra breath per week until you achieve a total of sixty. You can divide this into groups of fifteen, four times a day, or twenty morning, noon and evening, or thirty twice a day, whichever suits you best.

Relaxation exercises are equally important and here too we can follow Indra Devi's advice. To begin with, take off any jacket or shoes, and loosen your belt and tie if you are wearing them. If you wear glasses, put them aside. Now, lie down on the carpet and stretch. Stretch your arms way back over your head and stretch your legs, making the whole body as stiff as you can. Then, abruptly drop your hands down by your sides and relax the whole body. With your eyes closed, concentrate first on the tip of your toes and try to relax them. Imagine that your feet, legs and thighs are being gradually plunged into pleasantly warm water and all the muscles are becoming relaxed. Next, relax your back, spine and shoulders; then your arms, hands and fingertips. Let your chin drop so that the muscles of your face relax as well. And now, imagine that your body is getting heavier and heavier, so heavy that it sinks into the carpet and you no longer feel its weight. Remain like this for a few minutes – completely relaxed and completely at ease.

Now visualise yourself as a cloud – very light and carefree – just floating in the vast blue sky. After a while, dismiss this vision. Then try to keep your mind as blank as possible, but do not fight off intruding thoughts. Let them pass by and imagine yourself sinking into complete oblivion. To induce this feeling, try, with your eyes closed, to roll up your eyeballs and then lower them. You are relaxed, now, very relaxed, and feel like a light cloud floating in the sky. Before getting up, stretch and yawn. Turn on your right side and arch your back. Then repeat the same on the left side and stretch again. Lie down quietly for a moment. Finally, sit up, still yawning and stretching, and then slowly stand up – never jump up. How do you feel now? In those few minutes, didn't you relax as never before? And if you continue to do this every day, you will be able to break your tension and cast off your worries at will. A person who learns to relax learns the secret of a successful and healthy, long life.

As we mentioned earlier swimming is an excellent form of exercise for the body at all stages of life, and the water itself seems to bestow some extra benefit. Water treatments of any sort can be carried out very safely and efficiently, and even a simple bubble bath can be very soothing and effective. Dr Vogel – who was still skiing at the age of ninety-seven, was a great man for exercise and taught many women that if they wanted to keep as young and fit as possible after the age of fifty, underwater treatments – swimming followed by breathing exercises – were of great help, strengthening and toning the muscles and ligaments, as well as improving the circulatory system.

The next part of the chapter will explore many aspects of water and its therapeutic effects, even though some cannot strictly be described as exercise.

Several years have passed since I visited the headwaters of the Amazon River, but I still remember watching the natives bathe in the dirty waters of a tributary of the Maranon. In other tropical areas, I often saw the same thing: natives enjoying themselves in the muddy water, the water in some cases being absolutely black, in others more yellow or red. The Indians, and especially their children, would romp about in these dirty rivers without any fear of becoming sick as a result. They always seemed very happy and as if they were enjoying their dip. Despite the obviously good effect that a swim seemed to have on them, I never quite mustered enough courage to go in the water myself!

One day, however, I felt exceptionally tired and decided to try the inviting water. After all, the temperature was 40°C (105°F) in the shade and took a lot out of me after a while, especially as it was combined with an extremely high humidity. I had to keep reminding myself of the need to breathe deeply in order to cope a little better with the unbearable atmosphere. All I wanted was a refreshing bathe to bolster my spirits, but even so, I still did not have the courage to jump in the river. It then occurred to me that I could ask a local woman to fetch me some water in a large earthenware jug. I stood on a bamboo footbridge between two huts, and, as she brought the water, I poured it over my head, letting it run down all over me. The woman was kind enough to keep bringing one jug of water after another, and it was not long before I felt quite refreshed, even though the water was not as cool or as clean as I would have wished it to be.

Much later, I took a bath in a mud pond in the north of Scandinavia. When I stepped out of the muddy water, I felt completely refreshed. I then became curious about why this should be. It suddenly crossed my mind that we apply clay-water compresses because they are better than water packs. And then there are mud baths and the fango mud packs that are used as an application for sore areas and stiff joints; these too are judged to be more effective than simple water packs. It dawned on me that the muddy, that is, dirty, water was not that bad after all; I realised that it could still have a therapeutic effect in spite of its uninviting appearance, provided, of course, that the muddiness is nothing but natural dirt accounted for by clay or some other kind of earth.

On a later visit to the southwest USA, I came across a river – appropriately called Red River – that looked quite red. Such rivers derive their colour from red or yellow clay dissolved in the water; if they contain marshy soil, they become black as a result. Naturally coloured water is not necessarily unsuitable for bathing, but one has, of course, to be extra careful bathing in the tropics because of the abundance of parasites that pollute the streams. Just think of the dangerous schistosomes, liver flukes and micro-organisms galore, which transmit all kinds of dangerous disease.

I can well imagine that Father Sebastian Kneipp, the founder of hydrotherapy, would have been overjoyed if he could have seen such coloured river water; his natural instinct and intuition would have encouraged him immediately to investigate its medical effects. In fact, some time later an analytical chemist proved to me, by measuring the electrical tension in the water, that water carries energy that is transmitted to the human body. We filled a bathtub and then used the apparatus to measure the electric field in it. After the bath had been used, we measured its the electrical field once more and found that it had lessened, thus proving that the energy had been transmitted to the person bathing.

Not every kind of water, however, has the same electrical field, nor does it have the same therapeutic effect. The result depends upon the 'ballast' substances contained in the water, such as clay or black mud, which are responsible for the electrical charge. Minerals dissolved in the water can also add medicinal properties. These substances are usually picked up by the water as it flows from its source deep in the earth and on its way passes over mineral deposits. It is these substances which account for the remedial effects of water when used for bathing and drinking. Any colouring matter, which we at first consider to be impurities or dirt, will have been added to the spring water as it flowed over the deposits of clay and minerals. Thus, the therapeutic value, as well as the content of minerals and its energy or power, is produced in a natural way, which is of great importance.

As with inland rivers and streams, the sea too can have great therapeutic value. People who do not live by the sea dream of the beach and surf, especially when they sit down to plan their holidays. They long to see the play of the waves, how they break on the immovable rocks, roll, foam and then fizzle out on the golden sands. The waves approach the beach, powerful and inexorable, run up it and disappear, yet in spite of their awesome power they instil a feeling of being soothed. We never tire of watching them; we are just happy and content to admire their endless movement.

Bathing in the sea has various results. Salt water has an osmotic effect in that it draws water from the body. Therefore, those people who always have some excess fluid in the legs will feel considerably better after bathing in the sea. Sea water will do the same as sea salt packs would do. If you are overweight, sea-bathing will usually help you to lose weight, even though you may not eat less. This is because the sea stimulates the thyroid and gonads, thus benefitting the entire metabolism. All this is good for the figure, and slimness may then be within reach of some people. Sea air and sea-bathing are beneficial in cases of circulatory disorders, and diabetics will find swimming in the sea and walking over the sand good for them. Lazing around in the sun and heat is of no benefit to anyone: exercise during the day, plenty of rest at night and good food are what we need to make us feel fabulous.

When stress and tension threaten your health, do something about it quickly; take a holiday by the sea – there is no better remedy. However, while you are away from your work and duties, put them completely out of your mind and do not let the telephone interrupt your treatment. So, no telephone in your hotel room! 'Switching off' is absolutely essential during your holiday if you are to benefit fully from the 'cure' that the sea can give you.

There is one other rule that you must observe during your stay by the sea: go to bed early. That means that you must cut out any kind of night life and remember instead that the early morning hours are the best. In fact, after an early and restful night it is easier to wake up to go for a walk along the beach, feeling fully refreshed and fit. Remember, early to bed and early to rise makes a man (or woman) healthy and gloriously hungry for breakfast! What better ingredients could you have for this meal than a delicious fruit muesli, wholegrain or wholewheat bread with honey, and fruit or cereal coffee (Bambu Coffee substitute). The chapter on healthy eating can give you a few ideas on this.

But we can't necessarily nip off to the seaside when we feel a bit stressed, so we need a way to bring the benefits of hydrotherapy to us in our everyday lives, even if we cannot always set time aside for exercise in the form of swimming.

Alternating hot and cold water applications are excellent for poor circulation and a fine aid for removing any congestion. Apply hot water or herbal packs for about three minutes and then replace them by a cold water pack, leaving this on for no longer than half a minute. Repeat the hot pack, followed by the cold, and continue in the same way for twenty to thirty minutes. The same principle applies to water-treading. Tread your feet in hot water for three minutes, in cold water for half a minute, and so forth. If you take alternating hot and cold baths, you must stay in the cold water for only the same number of *seconds* as you were in the hot for *minutes*, as for alternating hot and cold foot and arm baths. These applications should never make you feel chilled – but always warm and comfortable.

Steam baths are useful for dispersing congestion, making the urine flow when retention occurs (older men often suffer from this difficulty) and relieving cystitis (inflammation of the bladder) and similar conditions of the bladder, as well as prostrate problems.

These baths are easy enough to prepare at home. First make a steaming hot infusion of hay flowers (using the stalks, leaves, blossoms, seeds and the hay itself), chamomile, wild thyme or similar aromatic herbs. When this is ready, pour it into a large vessel and place a narrow plank or board over it, on which you can sit. Keep the steam and heat from escaping by covering yourself from head to toe with towels or sheets. If you find sitting on the board uncomfortable, you can use a wicker chair instead, or you may be able to cut a hole out of the seat of an ordinary chair so that the steam can rise from underneath. In any event, you must keep your body warm and well wrapped in towels.

Keep adding more hot herbal infusion or hot water so that the steam continues to rise. This will be even more efficient if you can keep the infusion on a hot plate. Such a steam bath is very effective and inexpensive to construct, and serves an excellent purpose.

Sitz baths (in which only the hips and buttocks are immersed, hence their other name of hip baths) are part of good health care and, at the same time, complement effective beauty care. (See also the chapter on looking after your skin and hair.) If you take regular hip baths, the circulation will be stimulated, which, in turn, will benefit your abdominal organs. Did you know those external symptoms such as oily skin, blackheads, dandruff, skin eruptions and itchy skin can be the result of poor functioning of the abdominal organs? Such regular care and attention is especially good for the ovaries, since cold and congestion easily affect them which may alter a woman's emotional balance. Sitz baths increase blood circulation and eliminate stagnation, irritation and the initial stages of inflammation of the ovaries and fallopian tubes. Infertility can often be helped. A good circulation is also needed so that any natural remedies we take can reach the ailing parts of the body. Water therapies are the best treatments for this purpose, hip baths being most strongly indicated for women.

The addition of herbs, in the form of infusions, to the bathing water is highly recommended. For those who are nervous and tense, add lemon balm to the bath water. Dry and flaking skin benefits from an infusion of wild pansy (heartsease), while comfrey is good for rough skin with large pores. Another way to treat rough skin is to apply Symphosan (comfrey tincture) after every bath. If the skin is sensitive or sore, it is advisable to add an infusion of mallow (cheese plant) or sanicle. Oily skin responds well to herbal sea salt.

Hay flowers (hayseed) and juniper needles can also be added to a hip bath, as relaxants, and if you can obtain some eucalyptus leaves, these will have the same effect. Some of the aromatic herbs are stimulating, while others have sedative properties; you will have to make your choice according to the intended effect. Even oat straw can be a beneficial addition, although it is often considered useless as a medicine. Whatever the case, a hip bath is more efficacious when a herbal infusion is added: it would be a pity to take so much time and trouble preparing a Sitz bath if full use were not made of the herbs as remedies.

One of two hip baths should be taken every week, more when you are ill. The time spent in the bath may vary from twenty to thirty minutes, and the water must be kept at a constant 37°C (98.4°F – body temperature) which is accomplished by pouring some water off and replacing it with hot water. It is recommended that a hip bath be taken in the evening before going to bed, because you should not step out into the cold air afterwards or sit around in the house to cool off. A warm room is essential for such a bath as a cold room absorbs too much body heat. Additionally, it is advisable to wrap up well with warm towels; a reduction in body temperature or even beginning to feel chilly is detrimental when taking a bath.

The best vessel to use for a Sitz bath is, of course, one specially designed for that purpose; this will enable you to run off cooling water and add warm water, in order to maintain the required temperature. An ordinary bathtub will do, but you will have to keep a bucket of very hot water by the side of it. Use this hot water to top up the bath after removing some of the cooling water; to do this, you will need a jar and another bucket for disposal. If all you have is a bathtub, take a 'half bath', with the water reaching no higher than the navel. If you have both an ordinary bathtub and a small hip-bath, you can simply put a plank across the tub and stand the hip-bath on it. You will need another plank or board as a footrest. A hand shower attachment will make it quite easy to add more water, while the cooling water can be left to run into the unplugged bathtub underneath. The advantage of this arrangement is obvious: as well as being easier during the bath, the water can be emptied straight into the tub at the end of it.

Another form of hydrotherapy, the Schlenz method, uses baths of increasing temperature. In view of its many benefits, it is a method that deserves to be much more widely known and used.

I once met the old high school teacher Rudolf Schlenz in Innsbruck and shortly afterwards discussed the Schlenz method with his son, Dr J. Schlenz. My conversations with these two men conveyed to me some of the spirit of his wife, the late Maria Schlenz, who had developed this type of hot water therapy. Mrs Schlenz was neither a medical doctor nor a naturopath, but a simple housewife and mother. She had, however, an appreciation of nature and a gift for observation. In caring for her children, she realised that they were too delicate to benefit from Father Kneipp's cold water treatment, so she thought of giving them hot water treatments instead, followed by wrapping them up in hand-knitted woollen blankets. Some doctors had given baths of increasing temperature *(Uberwarmungsbäder)* with good results even before she began to use them, and continued to do so after the introduction of her method, but orthodox medicine in her native country paid no attention to her experience.

Later on, in Berlin, I made the acquaintance of Dr Devrient, one of those involved in the development of this treatment, who was so enthusiastic about the Schlenz method that he published a book explaining these baths, as well as sauna baths, as used in practice. He, along with Dr Walenski and Professor Lampert, was well known to Dr Vogel, and it is in this way that we know about the Schlenz method.

I learned about the regenerative and curative effects of hot water treatments used in Japan. The temperature of their baths surpasses that of blood temperature, and it is interesting to note that rheumatism and cancer are seldom heard of where these hot water baths are taken regularly. Some researchers even claim that swollen tissue can be rehabilitated if the water is kept 2–3°C above normal body temperature, i.e. at 39–40°C or 102–105°F. When the temperature is raised by 4–5°C, that is, up to 41–42°C (approximately 106°F), tumours are, according to these researchers, changed and in time dissolved. Many a malignant ailment can be prevented by their use, and the prevention of frightening diseases such as cancer has become a great necessity of our time. The prophylactic effect can help to maintain your health, but you must, of course, rouse yourself and apply your knowledge and the recommended treatment of a regular basis.

Increasing the body temperature by several degrees induces a kind of artificial fever, which is, just like a natural fever, able to burn up a lot of waste. I am reminded of a quote by Parmenides, the father of metaphysics: 'Give me the power to induce fever and I shall cure every illness.' Indeed, more healing can be done through increasing the body temperature than is generally thought possible. By raising the temperature to 40 or 41°C (approximately 105°F), disease-causing agents and tumour cells that are sensitive to heat will be destroyed. Those who suffer from metabolic and circulatory disorders will benefit greatly from a weekly Schlenz bath, as will anyone who has problems with their skin or lymphatic glands. It can also help to prevent the complications of multiple sclerosis.

Before you attempt a Schlenz bath in your home, you should first get to know the exact method as used in a recognised Schlenz bath centre, in order to enable you to become familiar with all the relevant details, although eventually bathing at home will obviously be more convenient and cheaper in the long run than hydrotherapy at a spa. The bathtub used for Schlenz baths is generally longer than an ordinary one and should preferably be made of wood. In modern homes, however, this is rarely the case, so a conventional enamel or plastic bathtub will do. It is also necessary to remember that your head will have to be immersed too, so you will have to bend your legs a little in a shorter tub.

Since the head is submerged too, the warmth will be equally distributed over the entire body, and congestion towards the head will be avoided. A Schlenz bath will therefore give no trouble at all, even though you may not be able to stand an ordinary hot bath. Keep the mouth and nose just out of the water so that you can breathe. As this position is uncomfortable and difficult to maintain for any length of time, attach a belt or a strong cloth at the top end of the bathtub to support the head. Reset the head on this support under the water, leaving only the mouth and nose in the air. To begin with, keep the water temperature at 36–37°C (97–99°F), that is, blood temperature, but be careful not to let the temperature drop. For this reason, it is important to have some hot water ready to add as necessary, letting the temperature rise to at least 38°C (100°F). Before taking the bath, drink one or two cups of hot herbal tea – lemon balm, peppermint, elder or goldenrod. Add a few drops of Crataegus if your heart is a little weak.

When you first start, a Schlenz bath should last only half an hour, but in time, you can increase the duration to two hours. In cases of obesity, it is advisable to add sea salt, brine or bath salt to the water, in addition to the herbs (see the section above on sea-bathing). An attendant should use a tough brush to vigorously brush down your entire body once or twice during the bath. This has the same effect as an underwater massage and stimulates the capillaries, thus removing congestion.

A Schlenz bath taken at home has the advantage in that you can go straight to bed and sleep. When the bath is over, sit upright, apply a little Po-Ho Oil (an oil that stimulates the sense of taste and smell), under your nose and inhale slowly, deeply and vigorously. As soon as the body has stopped perspiring, wash it down with lukewarm water and apply some St Johns wort oil to boost your spirits, either alone or in combination. Then stand up, wrap yourself in a warm bath towel and go straight into a warmed bed without drying yourself. You will continue to perspire while you are there. Your head and wet hair should be wrapped up warmly so that no part of your body can cool down. Then afterwards you will feel relaxed and pleasantly tired and will sleep soundly, waking fresh and energetic the next morning.

In contrast to this method, Louis Kuhne, a man with an astute mind and an understanding of natural healing, was able to use cold water treatment most effectively for what is called 'stimulation' or 'irritation' therapy. He perfected his method to such an extent that his handbook came to be translated into many languages, circulating to all parts of the globe. Unfortunately, he had no direct successor, so the Kuhne method is not as widely known as the cures developed by Priessnitz, Kneipp and other hydrotherapists.

Kuhne developed a cold water massage that is especially good for circulatory problems, such as cold feet. A simplified form of this treatment can be undertaken in your own home. First, take a large container and fill it three-quarters full with cold water. Then put a board over the container to cover half of it. Sit on the board, having taken off the clothes covering the lower part of your body. Take a brush with a long handle, wrap a cloth around the brush, dip it in the cold water and rub it round around your genitals. The cold reaction must only affect one part of the body, and for this reason your hand should not be put in the cold water but remain dry all the time. Because of the cold reaction, it is essential to maintain a constant body temperature by wrapping yourself in warm cloths or towels during the treatment, as is done during a steam bath.

In accordance with the body's reaction and the purpose for which it is intended, the treatment has to be undertaken for 10–15 minutes. However, always remember that you must not allow yourself to become chilled. Don't worry, you won't catch a cold from the cold water always being rubbed over the same area. This part of the body has an abundance of blood vessels and is therefore less sensitive to the cold. When massaging, avoid the region of the bladder because it is more sensitive.

The Kuhne treatment is best done at night to ensure restful sleep. It draws the blood from the head to the abdomen, with the effect that it is much easier to switch off distracting thoughts. If you find it difficult to go to sleep, you should try this method. Five minutes are often enough to draw the blood away from the head to the centre of the body, resulting in increased blood flow.

If your body does not respond to the cold water friction by making you feel warm, and you are quite sure that this is so, it would appear that the Kuhne method is not for you. If your body responds well to cold water applications, the Kuhne method will probably give you the desired results. These cold water friction or massage treatments relieve headaches, congestion in the head, fatigue, stomach upsets, loss of appetite and many other complaints. Frigidity as well as an exceptionally strong sexual drive can be treated successfully, so that in time it is possible to experience normal function of the sex organs. After a few weeks, cases of depression and melancholy can be improved, and these may even be cured if the treatment is continued over an extended period.

Having mentioned the potent effects of bathing in water, it is worth diverting for a moment to consider drinking water as you have to be even more careful with this. There are some wonderful spa waters available, but some also contain poisonous minerals, some of which I came across in North, Central and South America. It can happen that a stream may come from a mineral spring in which arsenic, copper or other heavy minerals are dissolved, making the water dangerous to drink. For this reason it is not possible to drink water from just any spring or source as one is able to do, in for example, Switzerland. It is often possible to recognise such dangerous springs by the discolouration of their rocks and stones or by sharp-tasting crystals in the river bed. Obviously, we should avoid these.

It is common knowledge that not all mineral waters have the same effect, and it would be foolish to ignore the fact that the mineral content of a certain water may be beneficial in the case of one particular illness but may not be so for another. Similarly, the same product doesn't help everyone. For example, those whose constitution is strong are more resistant to the effects, where as those who are more sensitive and weak always have to remember that although mild stimulation can be good, anything stronger may be harmful. So be careful. Volcanic areas with strongly radioactive springs can harm sensitive people and may even have a paralysing effect and endanger glandular function. If you become aware of an adverse reaction when staying in such places or taking the waters, it will be better to avoid them. On the other hand, do not forget that people of a stronger disposition and nature may benefit from a stay in a volcanic area; what may harm a weak person can possibly cure a stronger one. The simple rules are know your own limitations and weaknesses, keep your eyes open, and use only those things which are truly good for your health.

We have mentioned before how massage – a passive form of exercise – can be of great benefit, either alone or in combination with other therapies. Here, I will describe a method involving touch, which is related to this. The body seems to have a sixth sense, one which can be disturbing, especially as one grows older and it demands immediate attention and relief. It is a sense of intuition related to survival. Pain is a crucial element of this and should be attended to as soon as possible. Many chronic problems that cannot be alleviated or cured by your doctor or specialist can often be remedied by you yourself, using all forms of treatment – acupressure, acupuncture, osteopathy, chiropractice and so on. Basically, the power to heal your body lies within you – and you have the ability to achieve this by balancing the energies within your body. As discussed in earlier chapters, the energy within can be used to tremendous benefit in not only alleviating pain, but also balancing the body's energy system.

If we look at China, we see that thousands of men and women gain relief from pain and illness in several ways. There are doctors who have been trained to relieve and cure complaints by using certain energy points in the body. Traditional methods of treatment in Chinese medicine use needles, but even the fingertips alone can relieve pain and discomfort.

When asked about this sixth sense of pain, I feel that our intuition can play a leading role in directing us towards a suitable method of treatment. A number of hands-on techniques are very effective in relieving pain and discomfort. For example, place the tip of the index or second finger or thumb on the point where there is pain and, by giving this a little massage, immediate improvement can often be achieved; the body releases its natural painkilling substances – endorphins – when you do this. Or put your left hand over the painful area and place your right hand over it for a few seconds.

The illustrations below show thirty different 'healing' or 'energising' touches, to help to relieve pain, but also to help to balance the energy within, leaving you looking and feeling as fabulous as possible. By using these techniques of differing holds and touches, you are aiming to achieve bone symmetry within the area you are concentrating on. Study each of these thirty illustrations and you will form a firm basis for your healing and energising applications. You will be both pleased and surprised to discover how well these techniques work and, in particular, how good it feels to do these particular exercises.

But we mustn't forget our last form of exercise, that of mental exercise – exercising your mind and adopting a positive attitude, which we consider in the last two chapters of this book. Look in the mirror and see how beautiful you are. You have so many talents and so many qualities and attributes that other people do not – why not try to develop these, in a new hobby for example? Look carefully at your features and visualise the person you want to be; you will be surprised at the effectiveness of visualisation techniques. Bear in mind that you can be the happy, joyful, healthy, attractive and fabulous person you want to be.

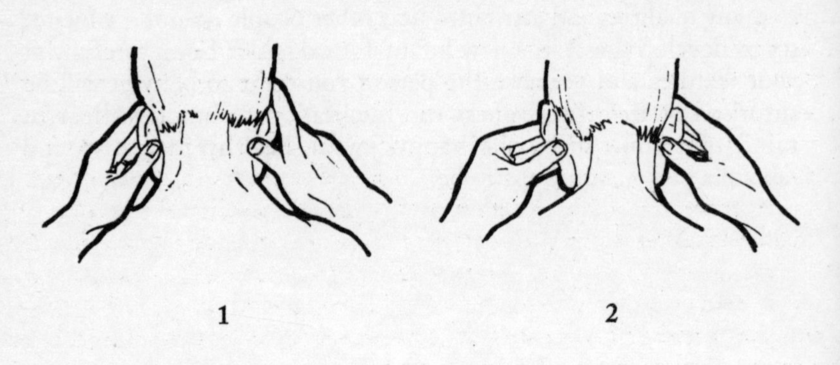

1

2

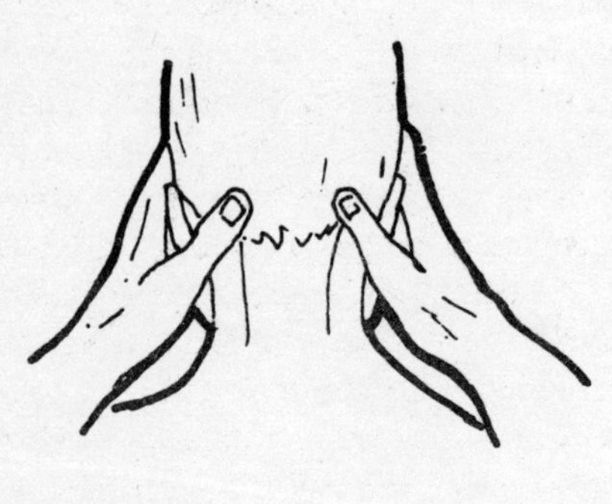

3

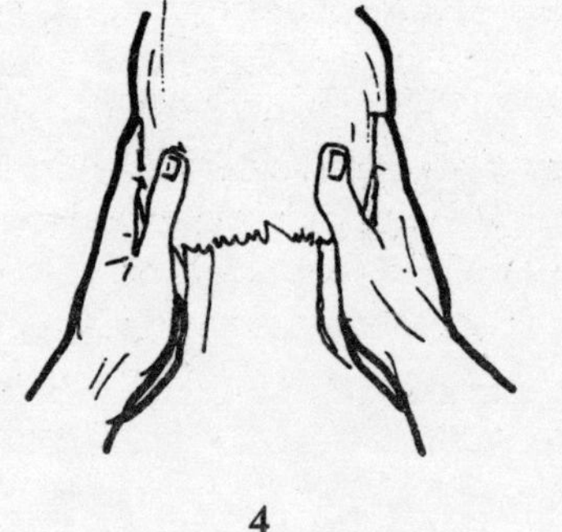

4

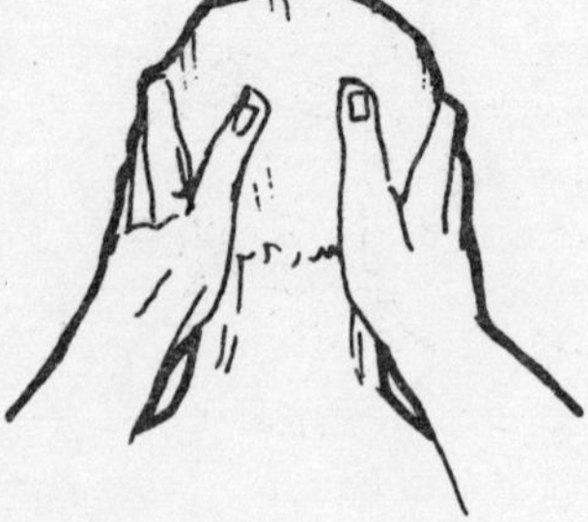

5

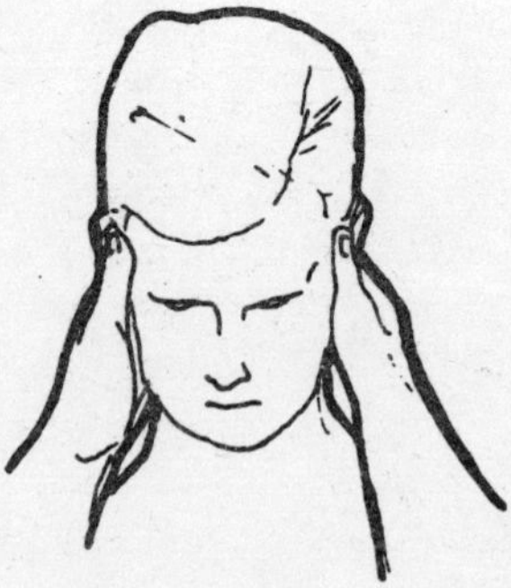

6

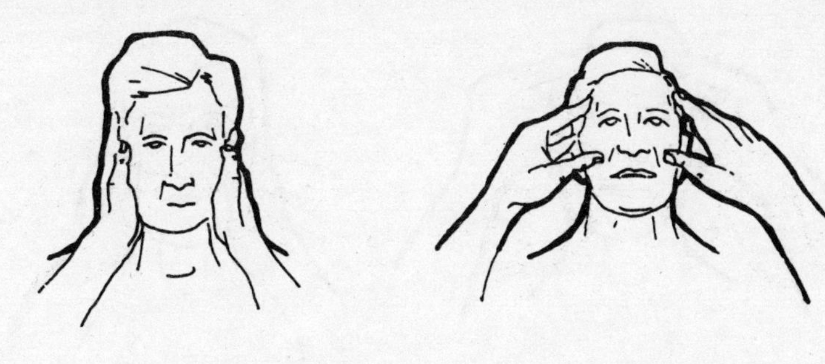

7

8

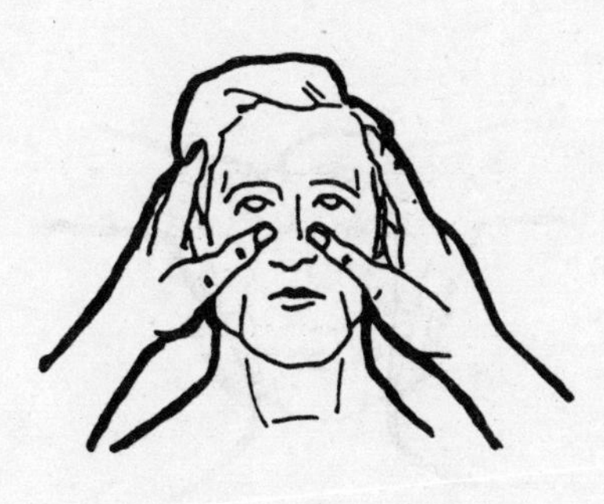

9

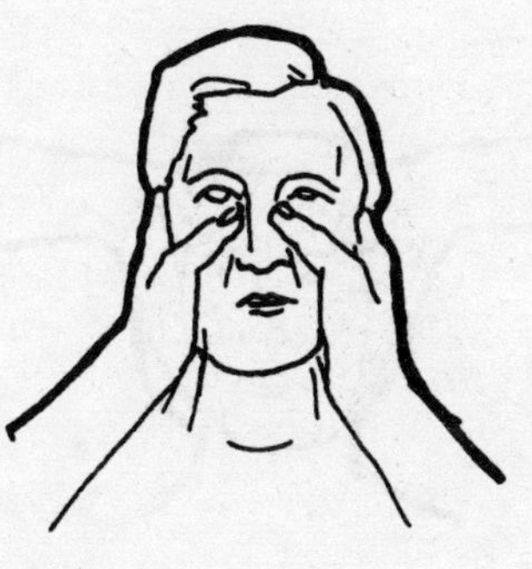

10

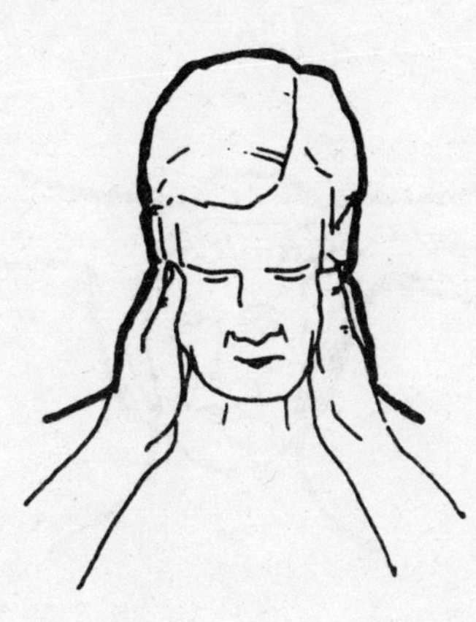

11

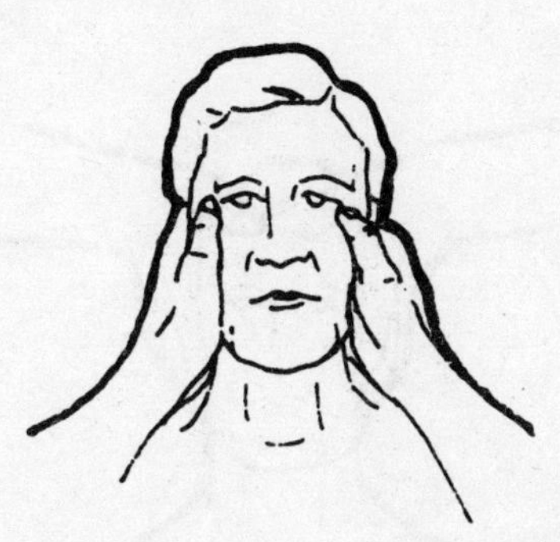

12

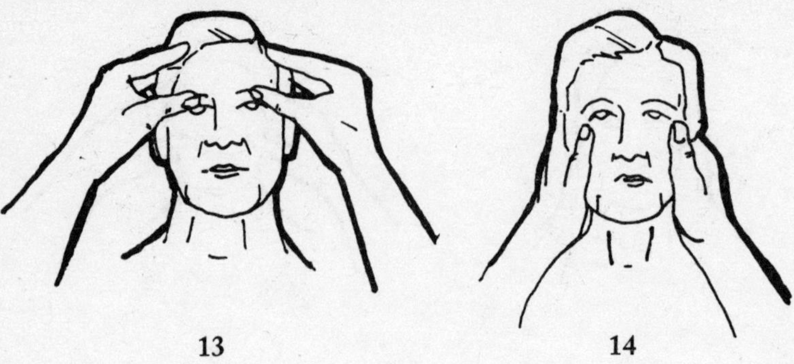

13

14

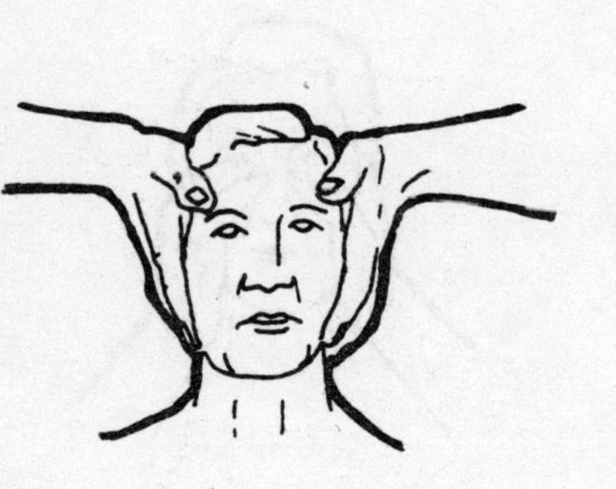

15

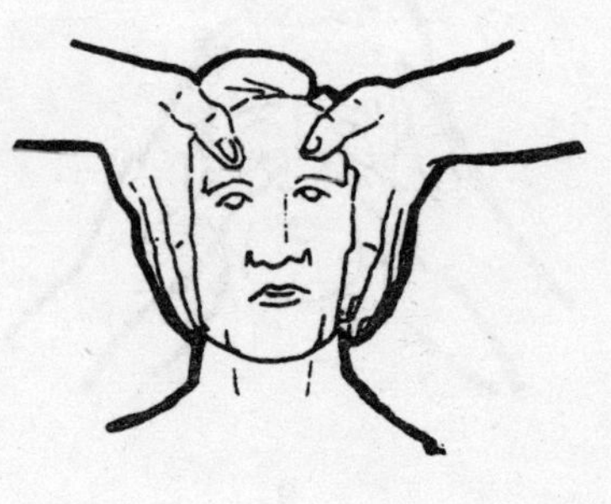

16

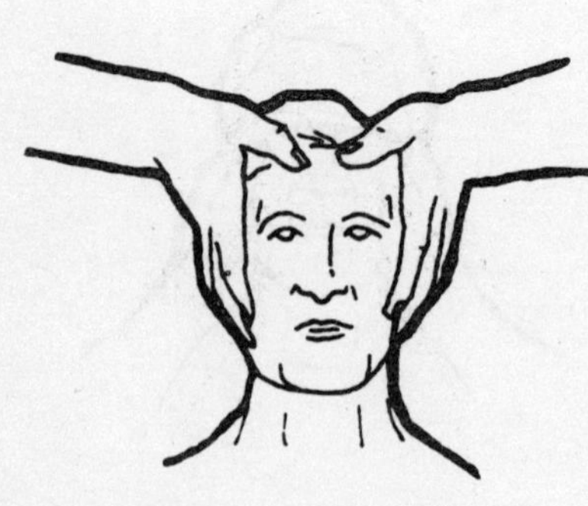

17

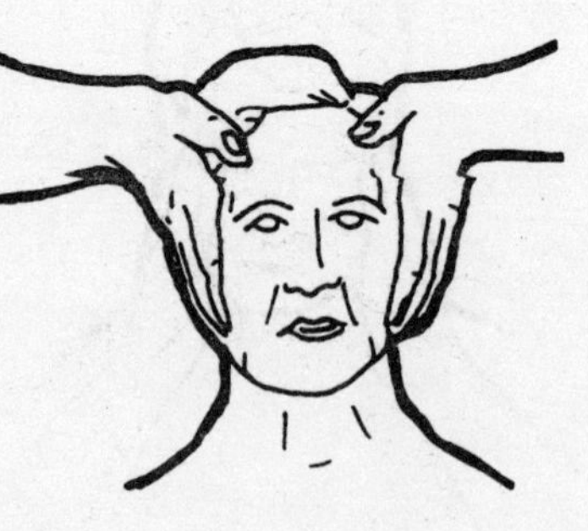

18

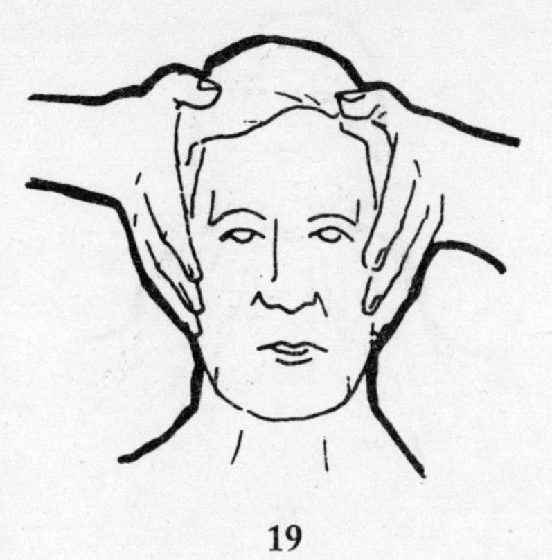

19

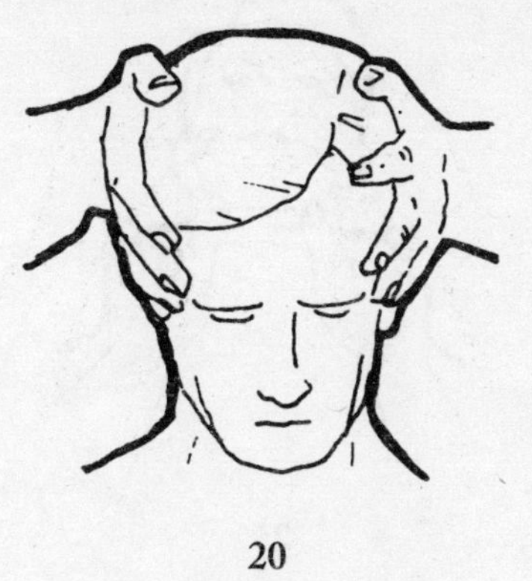

20

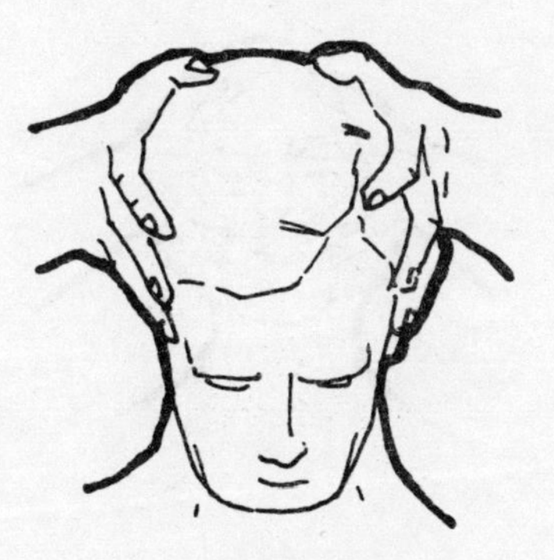

21

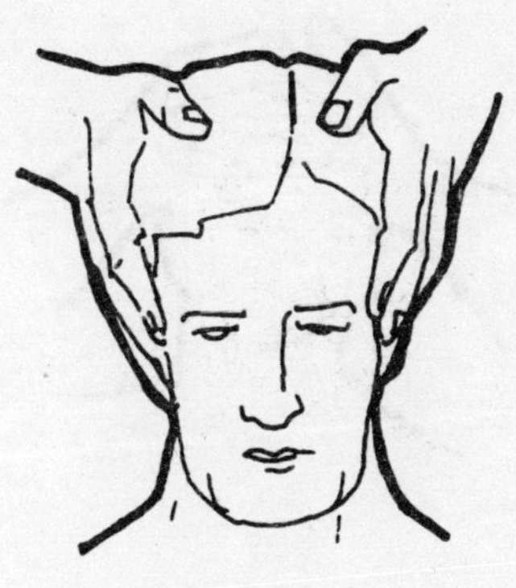

22

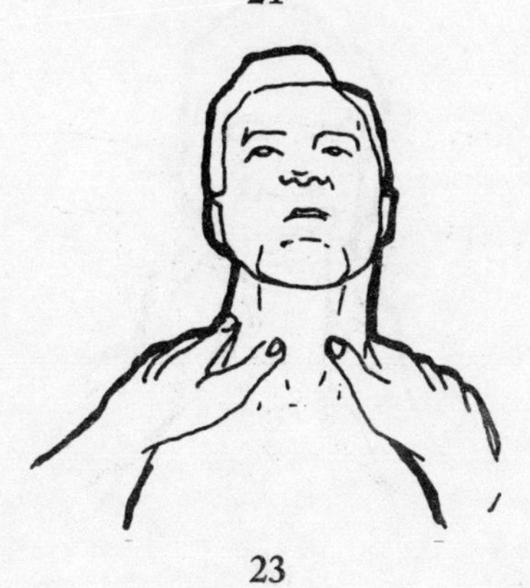

23

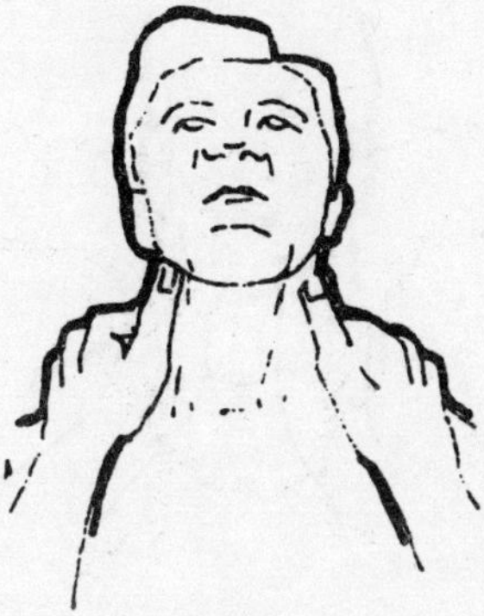

24

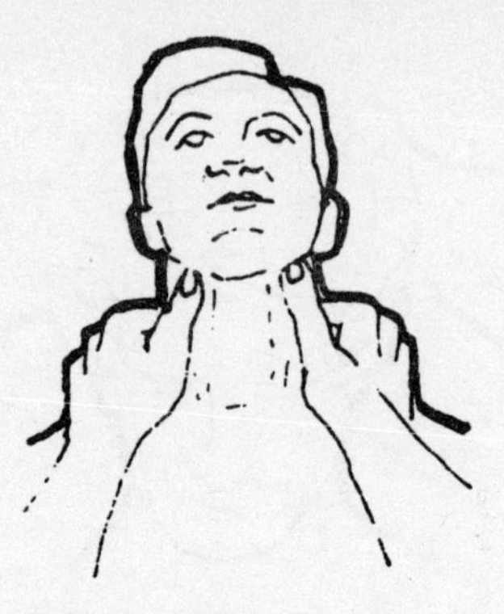
25

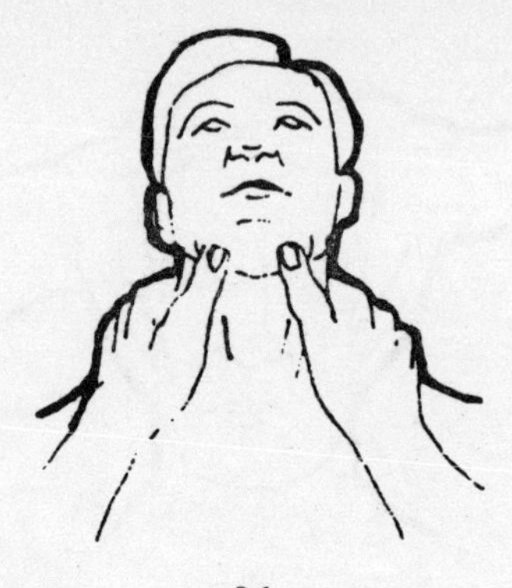
26

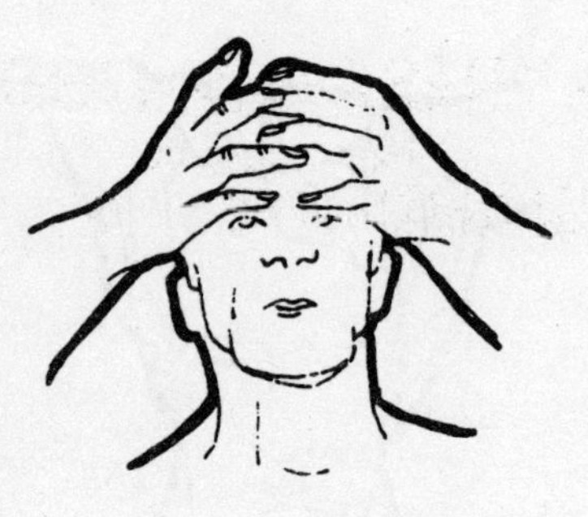
27

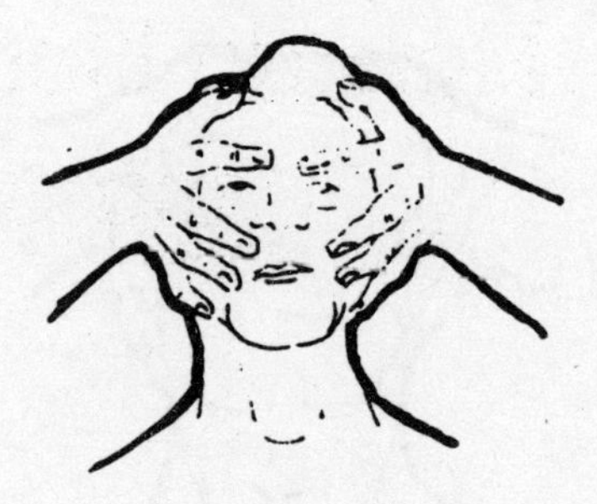
28

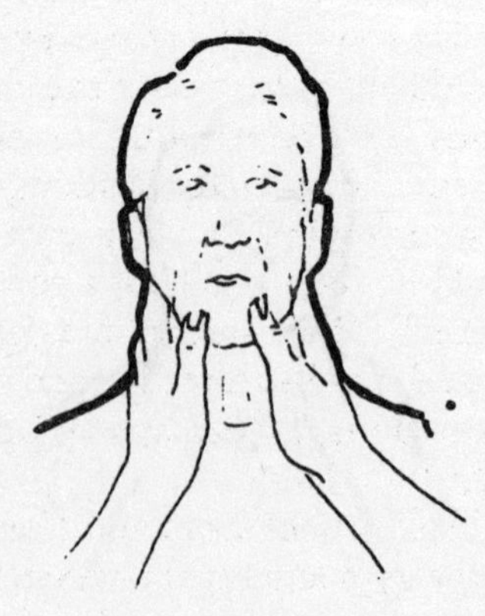
29

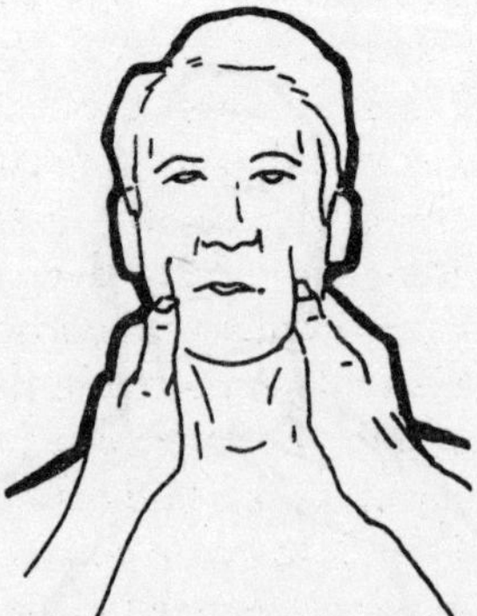

30

8

How do I look after my heart and circulation?

When my husband Stephen suffered a minor heart attack after only a few years of marriage, we learnt *together* how to deal with it and work to prevent a recurrence. Here are some of the things we learnt in practice that Jan will deal with in theory in the rest of the chapter.

The first aspect the heart specialist stressed was that the heart is a muscle and as such, needs to be exercised regularly. Walking is one of the best exercises – at least twenty minutes every other day, building up to forty-five. This should not be a stroll but a good firm walk. Swimming is another good exercise for heart patients because one is well supported in the water, and it is also a really good overall work-out. The type of exercise *not* to do is, for example, weights in the gym, as the body is being pushed too hard.

Well, I do go on the walks, but I still cannot swim and I certainly never was interested in weights in the gym anyway! However, where I *can* help Stephen is with his new diet; I am sure there can be nothing worse than looking at the other person across the table eating all the things that you are not allowed to.

What Stephen is 'permitted' certainly was an eye-opener. It seems ironic that it is only when a person is under pressure from an illness or condition that one hears from the doctor all the things he should and should not have: no dairy produce, no meat (certainly not lamb or pork), no shellfish (because of its cholestrol level). No alcohol of course (apart from the odd glass of red wine), but lots of fruit and veg, brown rice and pasta, oily fish and white meat. Apart from feeling better myself on this new regime, I feel that it must be helpful to one's partner join in and make sure this becomes part of a normal routine. Opposition or disinterest can only be of harm.

So whatever changes you make, they should become a new way of life, one that you work on together to improve your present and future health.

The old saying that you are as old as your circulation is highly appropriate, and circulatory problems are becoming an increasing worry nowadays. There are many people who experience difficulties with their circulation, for example women after the menopause, because they have not taken sufficient care and interest beforehand. With increasing age, we are more prone to damage to our blood vessels and hearts, so, in order to 'feel fabulous over fifty', we need to counteract this and, as much as possible, prevent further damage. Heart attacks, chilblains, osteoporosis, hearing problems, varicose veins and haemorrhoids are examples of conditions that have a link to the state of the circulation. Poor circulation also often has a knock-on effect on existing conditions. Osteoarthritis is one example – when the blood supply to the periphery becomes disrupted, the joint pain becomes more noticeable – and diabetes another. It is easy to think that this sort of thing only happens to other people, but after Gloria's experience, it is obvious that anyone is at risk.

In his book *The Nature Doctor*, Dr Vogel, who lived to a great age, gives excellent advice on looking after the circulation. He describes the function of the circulation by considering the analogy of the postal train travelling from Basel to Lugano and back, making stops right on schedule to unload on the way to Lugano, and picking up mail on the way back to Basel. Imagine the confusion if the train did not keep to its schedule – at each station, we can imagine the postmaster looking for the train and trying to calm the people who are waiting in vain for their letters to arrive.

Let us compare the train on its way to Lugano with the arterial network, which has the job of supplying the cells with nourishment to complete the process of feeding millions of cells. Minerals, vitamins, enzymes, amino acids, sugars, fats and oxygen are being transported by the arterial network to a strict schedule. Suppose that something interrupted the schedule and the cells failed to receive the various substances transported by the network, what would happen to the body? There would be a general breakdown, resulting in serious illness and possibly death. The more we learn of the individual function of different parts of the body like this, the more we can appreciate how wonderful are the works of the Creator.

Every little cell, like a factory, needs raw materials and fuel. If it is not supplied with all its needs on time during its lifespan, it cannot be expected to perform as efficiently. A lack of quantity and quality of raw materials forces the cells to find a makeshift solution, but it is only under the most trying conditions that the cells look for short cuts and thereby suffer in their performance. A case in point is shown by cancer cells. So we must, at all costs, ensure that the mail trains of our arterial system can keep to their schedules by stimulating our circulation through exercise and proper breathing techniques as described in the previous chapter. And above all, we must provide the raw material – from our food – at the proper time in sufficient quality and quantity.

So far we have spoken of only one function – one of construction; however, not only must supply be considered but, like every manufacturing plant, we must also concern ourselves with the waste products that the body produces. They must be promptly disposed of to enable the body to function efficiently.

The train on its way back to Basel can be compared to our venous system, which is responsible for returning all the 'ashes' and waste products, carbon dioxide, uric acids and so on. These waste products are recycled in the liver or eliminated with the help of the kidneys or lungs. If this process of transportation is obstructed, problems arise, since the accumulation of waste causes damage to all our tissues: the train may be derailed and the mail scattered everywhere.

When I think about the road traffic that passes incessantly every morning and evening along the highways leading to and from cities such as London and New York, I realise that the expression 'traffic arteries' is both justified and appropriate. If for some reason these arteries are paralysed, as they have been in the past from snow or torrential rain, the cities will also become paralysed. We too need free-flowing traffic in our arteries in order to survive. Even the most humanly perfect body, possessing a perfect muscular structure and well-organised bodily arterial traffic, will begin to decay or degenerate as soon as sclerosis or hardening of the arteries damages our intelligent, well-trained brain.

The anatomical structure of an artery is like that of a lagged pipe, made up of different layers, the inside one being a smooth tube. This arterial tube is covered with layers of tensile elastic, loosely woven threads. It can withstand a pressure of about 20 atmospheres (an atmosphere being a unit of pressure equal to 14.6 lb to the square inch) in order to withstand the force of the heart pumping into it.

The heart has its own feeding arteries, as do the arteries themselves, in this casc the so-called vasa vasorum, which are built into the inner walls of the arteries. Furthermore, the walls of the arteries have their own network of lymphatic vessels and nerves. The further removed the arteries are from the heart, the more branched out they become. To keep the total pressure within the system constant as the total cross-section becomes proportionally larger, the pressure in each falls, and the walls also become thinner. A capillary, the very finest vessel, is about 50 times less in cross-section than the finest human hair.

So we can see that anything that blocks or damages the arteries can have a very serious effect on any part of the body – the toes, the brain, the heart itself – depending where the blockage is. What could be responsible for such a problem? Factors include:

- a diet high in fats, especially animal fats – in red meat, butter and cheese, for example – which promotes an increased level of cholesterol in the blood, this eventually being deposited on the artery wall and narrowing the vessel
- nicotine from smoking is another extremely important factor contributing to a narrowing of the arteries, especially where the coronary vessels are concerned. The increase in the number of women smoking is thought to be one reason why heart attacks are being seen more in women

- a diet abundant in animal protein, such as that derived from meat, eggs and cheese
- too great a consumption of alcohol, which is harmful to the capillary walls and may thus contribute to the advancement of the disease. A glass of red wine a day is, however, thought to be, if anything, beneficial

These are all areas that we can alter, so even on the smallest scale, we can all make some lifestyle changes to improve our general circulation. The old saying 'prevention is better than cure' really does apply in this case.

The first area we will look at is that of blood cholesterol. Cholesterol, a type of fat, is transported in the blood on carrier molecules known as lipoproteins. The major categories of lipoproteins are very low-density lipoprotein (VLDL), low-density lipoprotein (LDL) and high-density lipoprotein (HDL). VLDL and LDL are responsible for transporting fats to the liver. Elevations of the level of either VLDL or LDL ('bad' cholesterol) in the blood are associated with an increased risk of developing atherosclerosis, the primary cause of a heart attack or stroke. In contrast, elevations of HDL ('good' cholesterol) are associated with a low risk of heart attack. It is currently recommended that the blood cholesterol level be less than 200 mg/dl, the LDL cholesterol level less than 130 mg/dl, the HDL cholesterol level greater than 35 mg/dl and the triglyceride (another type of blood fat) level less than 150 mg/dl.

So what about the ratio of the bad to the good cholesterol? The ratios of total cholesterol, and that of LDL, to HDL are referred to as cardiac risk factor ratios because they reflect whether cholesterol is being deposited into the tissues or broken down and excreted. The total cholesterol-to-HDL ratio should be no higher than four, and the LDL-to-HDL ratio should be no higher than 2.5. The risk of heart disease can be reduced dramatically by lowering the LDL cholesterol level while raising that of HDL. It has been concluded that for every 1 per cent drop in the LDL cholesterol level, the risk of a heart attack drops by 2 per cent. Similarly, for every 1 per cent increase in HDL level, the risk of a heart attack drops 3–4 per cent.

Although LDL cholesterol is often referred to as 'bad' cholesterol, an even more damaging form is lipoprotein(a) or Lp(a). A high level of Lp(a) has been shown to carry a ten times greater risk of heart disease than an elevated LDL cholesterol level as it sticks more easily to the walls of the artery. In fact, a high LDL cholesterol level carries less risk than a normal or even low LDL cholesterol level combined with a high Lp(a) level.

What, then, is the best way to lower the cholesterol level? The most important approach to lowering high cholesterol is a healthy diet and lifestyle. The dietary guidelines are straightforward: eat less saturated fat and cholesterol by reducing or eliminating animal products in the diet, increase the consumption of fibre-rich plants foods (fruits, vegetables, grains and pulses), and lose weight if necessary. Lifestyle factors include getting regular exercise, not smoking, and reducing or eliminating the consumption of coffee (both caffeinated and decaffeinated).

In many cases, however, diet is not sufficient to lower the cholesterol level. Fortunately, there are several natural compounds that can lower the cholesterol level and other significant risk factors for coronary artery disease. In fact, when all the factors (cost, safety, effectiveness) are considered, the natural alternatives that I will discuss below offer significant advantages to standard drug therapy.

Because of its low cost and proven efficacy, my first recommendation is to try niacin (vitamin B), whose cholesterol-lowering activity was first described in the 1950s. The side-effects of niacin described below can be avoided by using a special form of niacin known as inositol hexaniacinate, or hexaniacin. Niacin has been shown to lower the levels of LDL cholesterol, Lp(a) triglyceride and fibrinogen (which is involved in blood clotting) while simultaneously raising the HDL cholesterol level. Its use has been shown in trials to reduce overall mortality. In a comparison with lovastatin, one of the new lipid-lowering drugs, it has been shown that while lovastatin produced a greater effect on LDL cholesterol reduction, niacin provided better overall results despite the fact that fewer patients were able to tolerate a full dosage of niacin because of skin flushing. The percentage increase in HDL cholesterol, a more significant indicator for coronary heart disease, was dramatically in favour of niacin. Equally impressive was the percentage decrease in Lp(a) seen with niacin.

Niacin does, however, have some side-effects. The most common and bothersome is that of skin flushing, which typically occurs twenty to thirty minutes after the niacin is taken. Other occasional side-effects of niacin include gastric irritation, nausea and liver damage. In an attempt to combat the acute reaction of skin flushing, several manufacturers have begun marketing sustained-release, time-release or slow-release niacin products, which allow the niacin to be absorbed gradually. However, while these forms of niacin reduce skin flushing they have proved to be more toxic to the liver and less easy for patients to tolerate. Indeed, it has been strongly recommended that the use of sustained-release niacin be restricted because of the high percentage (78 per cent) of patient withdrawals as a result of side-effects.

Because niacin can impair glucose tolerance, it should be used with close observation in patients with diabetes. Niacin should not be used in patients with pre-existing liver disease or an elevation in liver enzymes; these groups should instead take gugulipid, garlic or pantethine. For some reason, non-diabetic patients may not respond to niacin, so for them too I recommend gugulipid, the standardised extract of the mukul myrrh tree (*Commiphora mukul*), native to India.

Several clinical studies have confirmed that gugulipid has an ability has an ability to lower both cholesterol and triglyceride levels by up to 30 per cent, also increasing the HDL level by up to 20 per cent. The dosage of gugulipid is based on its content of guggulsterone, the active ingredient. Clinical studies have demonstrated that gugulipid extract standardised to contain 25mg of guggulsterone per 500 mg tablet, given three times per day, is an effective treatment. No significant side-effects have been reported with purified gugulipid preparations, but crude guggul preparations such as gum guggul are associated with, for example, skin rashes and diarrhoea. Thus you must ensure that you are using the purified standardised extract.

In diabetics, I typically recommend pantethine over inositol hexaniacinate. Pantethine is the active form of vitamin B5, or pantothenic acid. For some reason, it has a significant lipid-lowering activity while pantothenic acid has very little (if any) effect on the cholesterol and triglyceride levels. Pantethine's mechanism of action is by inhibiting cholesterol synthesis and accelerating the utilisation of fat as an energy source. Pantethine administration has been shown significantly to reduce serum triglyceride, total cholesterol and LDL cholesterol levels while increasing that of HDL cholesterol. These effects become even more impressive when its virtually lack of toxicity is compared with that of conventional lipid-lowering drugs.

The safest form of niacin at present is inositol hexaniacinate. It yields slightly better results than standard niacin, but is much better tolerated, both in terms of flushing and, more importantly, long-term side-effects. Regardless of the form of niacin being used, periodic (for example, every three months) checking of the cholesterol level and liver function tests is indicated.

Sustained release niacin should not be used. If pure crystalline niacin is used, start with 100 mg three times a day and carefully increase the dosage over a period of four to six weeks to the full therapeutic dose of 1.5–3 g daily in a divided dose. If inositol hexaniacinate is used, begin with 500 mg three times daily for two weeks and then increase to 1000 mg. Crystalline niacin and inositol hexaniacinate are best taken with meals.

Although this usually produces a significant fall in the cholesterol level within the first two months, those with an initial cholesterol level of over 300 mg/dl may need to wait four to six months before the cholesterol level begins to reach normal. Once a patient's cholesterol level falls below 300 mg/dl, reduce the dosage of niacin to 500 mg three times daily for two months. If the cholesterol level then creeps above 200 mg/dl, the dosage of niacin can be raised to 1000 mg three times daily. If the cholesterol level remains below this, however, the niacin can be completely withdrawn and the cholesterol level rechecked in two months, niacin therapy being reinstituted if it has crept above 200 mg/dl.

Anyone with a high cholesterol level should also take a garlic supplement. Clinical research recommends that a commercial garlic product should provide a daily dose of 10 mg of alliin, or a total allicin (potential yield) of at least 4000 μg. It has been concluded in expert reviews that the anti-atherosclerotic effects of garlic are derived from the constituents of alliin and allicin, so preparations standardised for these provide the great assurance of quality and results.

Having aimed to improve our cholesterol level, can we tell how efficient our circulation is? We can get some clue from how we respond to seasonal changes. Whatever our age, few of us are unaffected by this; some are fortunate enough to suffer from cold hands and feet alone, but for others it can be the beginning of a miserable and painful few months as the result of chilblains arising from a poor circulation. As a simple test, gently squeeze your nail. The colour should return to your fingernail immediately you let go. If it doesn't you may like to try some circulation-boosting methods, using diet, herbs, hydrotherapy, exercise and massage. We will look at these below, and you might also like to read earlier chapters in this book, which go into these topics in more detail.

A few very basic changes can also be made. Sensible clothing is most important in winter; the abdomen, legs, hands and feet should be covered sufficiently to ensure warmth, and high heels should definitely be avoided as they throw the whole body out of balance. Some people may be able to change their occupation or delegate part of their work in order to avoid prolonged endurance, especially in cold and damp environments, and this is always worth considering.

As we mentioned in a previous chapter, try to adopt a diet that is low in salt and saturated (animal) fats and high in fruit and vegetables. Surprisingly, as Gloria recently discovered, shellfish are one of the worst foods for raising one's cholesterol level. There is no substitute for a balanced diet of fresh foods – good food does not come out of a packet or a tin, and anything that has a shelf life of longer than a couple of years cannot be healthy. Just look at your fruit bowl or salad tray after a week to see how fruit and vegetables go off in their natural state. Gloria recently attended a very exhilarating meeting on the power of diet in preventing coronary heart disease and will describe it here.

The most recent example of prevention, and taking your health into your own hands, comes from America following fifty scientific studies showing that eating whole grain as part of a balanced and healthy diet can reduce the risk of heart disase and certain cancers by up to 30 per cent.

For example, one study of over 75,000 women found that those consuming the most whole grain had a 30 per cent lower risk of coronary heart disease than the group consuming the least. Another study involving 34,000 women found that whole grain intake reduced the risk of death from heart disease. Those eating one or more servings per day had a 40 per cent reduction in total mortality over nine years. This was a particularly detailed study over a substantial period of time, so its findings an be taken as valid.

So what exactly is classified as whole grain? It simply means that *all* parts of the grain are used: fibre-rich bran (the outer layer), the endosperm (the middle layer) and the nutrient-packed germ (inner layer). These whole grains are packed with nutrients that are essential for good health. It was previously thought that the whole grain reduced the risk of disease because it is such a good source of fibre, but this latest research confirms that components such as antioxidants, vitamins, minerals, complex carbohydrates and phytonutrients, which protect the body against many diseases, are also involved.

When a survey was carried out in Britain, there was much confusion regarding what whole grain actually is: 75 per cent did not know what at all, 67 per cent thought all cereals were whole grain, and 65 per cent thought that all breads were whole grain. Many thought that if a foodstuff were 'brown', it had to be whole grain. Most people knew the value of grains for bowel movement, but only 4 per cent knew of the other benefits of using whole grain.

Whole grain can be whole grain oats, whole grain rice, whole grain rye or whole grain wheat. The recommendation is to have three portions of whole grain each day, which is actually very easy to introduce. This can be taken as a cereal or porridge for breakfast, for example, a good healthy sandwich made from whole grain bread at lunchtime, and a whole grain pasta or rice in the evening. When shopping at the supermarket, check the label to see whether whole grain comes top of the list of the ingredients. Further information can be obtained from 'Whole grain for health' on 020 7331 5445.

It seems incredible that such simple changes can have such significant health benefits. So the message must be 'Go with the grain'.

In summary, make an effort to begin cooking and preparing your own food for the bulk of your diet and eat more natural and fresh foods.

The plant kingdom has plenty to offer to keep the body running smoothly. Certain berry and flower extracts, for example of chamomile, rosemary and mistletoe, have powerful blood pressure-lowering effects and can even improve the symptoms of angina. Herbal medicine can be of great help in stimulating and maintaining a healthy heart and circulation. Many herbs have been used safely in traditional and folk medicine, and they are now making a comeback as the natural remedy of choice in the treatment of circulatory problems.

Women in particular can benefit from a well-known revitalising remedy consisting of the four herbs milfoil, St Johns wort, (*Hypericum perforatum*), arnica root and pulsatilla. An extract of horse chestnut, in addition to the above herbs, is a natural aid to body function. As mineral deficiencies also contribute to the formation of varicose veins, a calcium complex should be taken to ensure successful treatment. If we support our circulatory organs sensibly and naturally, pain and discomfort may be avoided later.

Cayenne pepper, meanwhile, is well known to cooks, but its effect on the peripheral circulation – that which flows to the extremities – is less well known. Taken as a herbal medicine, cayenne can boost the blood supply to the chilly corners of the body – just the remedy for cold winter evenings, or for those with eternally cold feet or hands. A light dusting of cayenne pepper on the affected areas will stimulate the local circulation.

Hawthorn (*Crataegus oxyacantha*) has profound effects on the heart, supporting its efficiency as a pump and regulating its beat. It can be considered to be a natural alternative to digoxin, the drug most commonly prescribed for heart failure. The berries and flowers of the hawthorn are very concentrated sources of plant-based chemicals known as anthocyanidins and proanthocyanidins, which give the berries their colour. These phytochemicals can increase the absorption of vitamin C and, at the same time, strengthen the walls of the small blood vessels and capillaries. The blood cholesterol level is also reduced, further supporting hawthorn's special place in natural heart care.

As with many herbs, the exact mechanism behind the plant's action on the heart and circulation is not fully understood – but what is known is that the drop in blood pressure that it produces appears to be caused by an opening up of the larger blood vessels. This interesting herb is also a good example of how natural therapeutic agents work better when taken as a whole rather than as a highly purified extract; another example is that of mistletoe.

When mistletoe's ability to lower blood pressure was first noted, scientists rapidly separated its chemicals out and started testing them one by one. To the astonishment of the research team looking at the herb, the blood pressure-lowering effect could not be replicated until they used the whole plant tincture. It appeared that the various biologically active substances acted together to produce the final result, but taken individually, they had no effect. This experiment beautifully supports the concept of holistic medicine.

Mistletoe is commonly combined with other herbs. Care must be taken, however, when self-prescribing as it is potentially very toxic, so always seek the advice of a naturopath or herbal practitioner experienced in using this herb.

Most people know from the popular press that garlic is good for them, but the smell tends to put many people off taking an effective daily dose. Garlic has been studied in great depth: there is in fact an International Society for the Study of Garlic, which encourages scientists from around the world annually to pool their collective knowledge. Most research has focused on the herb's ability to lower blood cholesterol, but a good deal of work has been done on its ability to lower blood pressure. This can be quite significant, causing a fall of up to 30 mmHg in the systolic (the top value in a blood pressure measurement) and by up to 20 mmHg in the diastolic (the lower value in a blood pressure measurement) reading. Onions have a similar effect.

It is probably worth digressing for a moment to look at blood pressure. This is simply the pressure exerted by the blood on the walls of the vessels through which it travels. As we can guess from the section above where we described the blood vessels, the pressure varies round the system, as well as with whether the heart is pumping the blood out or relaxing to collect the blood coming back from the body.

So that we can have a universal system on which to base our knowledge of health and treatment, the blood pressure measured is always that in the arteries, usually in the arm. The higher reading (the systolic pressure) reflects the heart pumping out. Its value increases with age and varies between individuals but should, as a very rough guide, be lower than 100 plus your age.

The lower (diastolic) value occurs when the heart is collecting the blood back in. Again it increases with age, but should be below about 90 mmHg for health. The higher either blood pressure reading goes, the more at risk we are of, for example, a heart attack or a stroke. One easy way to lower your blood pressure if you are overweight is to lose weight. Raised blood pressure is medically known as hypertension.

Some say that low blood pressure is never a problem, but this is not actually the case. Low blood pressure (hypotension; less than about 110/70 mmHg) is an interesting condition because it is not officially recognised by the UK medical profession. In Germany, however, it is a common diagnosis and is treated with the same seriousness and care as high blood pressure (hypertension).

Garlic is also one of nature's best anticoagulants, helping to prevent the blood clotting in the vessels themselves. If bits (thrombi) break off these clots, they can travel round the body and get stuck in any of the smaller vessels. It is particularly dangerous if this happens in the heart, lungs or brain as this can cause a heart attack, a stroke or even death. A daily dose of garlic is a natural way to counteract this.

Boosting the circulation, especially that to the brain, is of prime importance as one gets older. The best remedy for this is *Gingko biloba* extract, a strong and useful preparation. This is one of the longest-known and safest products on the market to boost an inefficient circulation. The *Ginkgo biloba* tree is the world's oldest living tree species and can survive as long as 1000 years, growing up to a height of more than 30 m (100 feet). Extracts from the leaves of the ginkgo tree are used medicinally and have been studied extensively in Europe, now being among the leading prescription medicines in both Germany and France. Extracts identical to these preparations are available in the USA and Canada as food supplements.

The active components of the ginkgo leaves are the gingko flavone glycosides or gingko heterosides. The most effective and widely studied form of gingko is an extract of the leaves standardised to contain 24 per cent ginkgo heteroside. Interestingly, the total extract is more active than its single isolated active ingredient. This suggests a synergism between the various components of the Ginkgo biloba mixture – an explanation that is well supported by more than three hundred clinical and experimental studies utilising it.

The primary clinical application of gingko extracts has been in the treatment of vascular insufficiency, but it is most commonly thought of as a powerful herb for the brain, as it improves memory and other brain functions by enhancing blood flow to the brain. It has been used medically for cerebrovascular insufficiency and impaired mental performance, Alzheimer's disease, cochlear (inner ear) deafness, senile macular degeneration and diabetic retinopathy – conditions affecting the vision – impotence, premenstrual syndrome, depression, allergies and asthma.

Experimental studies as well as preliminary clinical evidence indicate that *Ginkgo biloba* extract may also be of benefit in cases of angina, congestive heart failure and acute respiratory distress syndrome and it may additionally have a role in the treatment of conditions such as various types of stroke, thrombosis, graft protection during organ transplantation, multiple sclerosis and burns.

Make sure the gingko product you use has the standardised extract containing 24 per cent gingko heterosides clearly described on the label. The recommended dosage is 40 mg of this standardised product three times daily although some studies have used a slightly higher dosage of 80 mg three times daily. It is difficult to determine the dosage of non-standardised products as there is such a variation of active content. Clinical research clearly shows that *Gingko biloba* extract should be taken consistently for at least 12 weeks in order to be effective. Although most people report a benefit within two or three weeks, some may take longer to respond.

Gingko biloba extract is extremely safe and side-effects are extremely uncommon. In contrast to the tolerance of the leaf extract, contact with or ingestion of the fruit pulp has been reported to cause severe gastrointestinal irritation.

Another very effective preparation for improving the circulation is vitamin E, which Gloria takes daily. In addition, there is a new Dutch remedy called Elastovas, which I formulated with the company Enzypharm in Holland and can be obtained from SHP; it is one of the finest remedies that I have come across in resolving arterial problems. Elastovas, which contains amino acids and plant enzymes, can be taken at a dose of fifteen drops, in half a glass of water, twice a day. My oldest patient, who is 104, takes this remedy, enjoys a clear healthy mind and, as she herself says, feels fabulous!

Daily exercise, even if it is just a daily walk, is one of the most effective ways to boost your circulation. As well as toning up the heart, the muscular activity pumps the blood in the veins back towards the heart and stops it pooling in the extremities. Exercise is important, even if you suffer from high blood pressure: walking, gentle swimming and cycling will all help reduce this. This may sound odd since, in any exercise programme, the heart will be stimulated, but the long-term effect of aerobic-style exercise is a lowering of the blood pressure. If you are worried it is advisable, as always, to seek professional advice.

Massage can be of great help to people suffering from symptoms of a sluggish circulation, and essential oils, as used in aromatherapy, can also be applied to further enhance the effect of the massage. Aromatherapy plays an important role in stimulating blood flow and can be helpful to people suffering from the symptoms of a sluggish circulatory system. When dealing with a poor circulation, combining essential oils with regular massage often proves to be the most effective way of using them as both bring oxygen and other nutrients to relevant area and help to remove carbon dioxide and other waste material to the lymphatic system, from where it will be passed out of the body.

There are three basic aromatherapy massage movements that can be used to stimulate the circulation. The long stroking movement is the most common and well-known technique. This is called effleurage and is used not only at the beginning and end of a massage, but also in between other movements. It is ideal for spreading the oil, but its main purpose is to stimulate the circulation. This technique is also used for relaxation purposes, and when giving massage, it is important to start with light strokes, slowly increasing the pressure.

Spreading movements are important for the release of muscular tightness but are also used to improve the circulation. These movements are firm, squeezing techniques whereby the skin and surface muscle are squeezed and rolled.

One of the most beneficial techniques for poor circulation is that of friction movements. These are warming and stimulating circular movements. Again, the depth of the technique can be varied. None of these techniques should be painful. Although a general massage can be given by someone else to improve your general circulation, it is not really necessary as you can easily do it yourself. If you want to improve your circulation, massage your hands and feet daily.

For a simple foot massage, stroke the foot from the toes to the heel to spread the oil. Then move onto the arch of the foot and, with gentle movements of the thumbs and fingertips, slowly work towards the soles and the sides of the foot using the palm of the hand. Then stroke the base of the foot from the toes to the heel and repeat the kneading from the arch to the side of your foot. Bend each toe and then squeeze the foot rhythmically; finish by stroking the base of the foot.

Move onto the calves using long stroking movements. Start at the heel and use the palms of both of the hands to glide up the back of the calves. Then slowly knead the calf muscles using your fingers and finish by stroking upwards with alternate hands before moving to the front of the leg. Again, apply the same upward stroking movements using one hand at a time. With your fingertips, trace gentle circular movements around the knee and then apply the same long upward sweeping movements to the upper thigh, first at the front and then at the back of the thigh. Finally, move onto the other foot and leg.

Massage of the hands is just as quick and easy. Spread the oil onto the palm of the right hand using the left hand. Then gently knead the palm of the right hand using the thumb of the left hand. Work around the palm towards the fingertips and then gently pull each finger, finishing by using the stroking action again. Turn your hands over and apply the oil to the back of the right hand using the left. Then stroke from the fingers, across the back of the hand and up your arm to the elbow. Repeat this a couple of times. Turn your arm over, and use the same long stroking movements up the inside of the arm to the elbow. Then, using one thumb and finger, knead the muscles of the forearm to the elbow and finish again with long effleurage movements from the hand to the elbow. Repeat the procedure on your other hand and arm.

Many oils can be used to benefit a sluggish circulation, the most effective being those which provide a warming effect, such as cypress, yarrow, rosemary and lemon. These stimulate the local blood flow and bring heat to the surface of the skin. Essential oils, with a couple of exceptions, cannot be applied directly to the skin, so a few drops of your chosen oil needs to be mixed with a carrier oil such as vegetable, almond, wheatgerm or even avocado oil, for example 30 drops of your chosen oil with 30 ml of carrier oil. Alternatively, try adding a few drops of the oil mixture to your bath.

If you have a home blood pressure test kit, try taking your blood pressure before and after an aromatherapy massage using either juniper or melissa oil; you may be pleasantly surprised at what you find. There is, however, one word of warning: certain essential oils, including hyssop, rosemary, sage and thyme, can aggravate high blood pressure and should thus be avoided.

Anyone who has suffered from muscular rheumatism, joint stiffness or the symptoms of arthritis will enjoy a soothing massage. Stimulation of the local circulation and the dispersal of toxins that collect in and around the joint and muscle in response to injury or chronic inflammation can have an almost immediate effect on the health of the tissues. To promote the elimination of toxic matter, try adding fennel, lemon, juniper or lovage oil to your carrier oil.

This simple oil-based massage can be improved upon with the introduction of oils with rubefacient (warming) effects. Camphor, eucalyptus and pine have been used for this purpose for centuries, and often form the basis of expensive over-the-counter preparations marketed for the relief of muscular aches and joint pains; it is possible to make up your own oil combination at home that is just as effective as the ready-made proprietary brands.

Gentle drainage massage can be helpful for water retention (oedema) which is commonly experienced by premenopausal women in the time leading up to the menstrual period and those with high blood pressure. The key symptoms are swelling of the ankles and, premenstrually, breast tenderness. Always direct the massage strokes towards the nearest lymphatic junction. For the ankles and calf, this is found at the back of the knee, whereas for the breast tissue, the armpit is the point of drainage. Try applying the drainage massage after a warm bath so that the circulation is pre-stimulated and tissue fluid exchange is already occurring.

A slowing of the circulation (venous stasis), combined with the effects of gravity, appears to lie behind the common problem of varicose veins. This occurs when the blood cannot get back to the heart quickly enough. A congestive problem occurs because as more blood continues to arrive, it collects behind the blood that is trying to make its way back to the heart. As the pressure increases, the valve in the vein distends as it buckles under the high back-pressure. Unlike arteries, veins have thin walls, so these sag and a characteristic bulge can be seen and felt. A stimulation of the general circulation is needed, but gentle local massage that encourages circulation and drainage of the congested vein is very beneficial.

Hydrotherapy has also been used for many centuries to stimulate sluggish circulation. An easy way to do this is using a shower, alternating from hot to cold water, and always finishing with the cold. The fluctuation in temperature has a pumping effect on the circulation: the cold water will reduce the peripheral blood flow by constricting the blood vessels and the hot water will increase it by dilating them. If you cannot face treating your whole body, try your feet first and then your legs. Perhaps, one day you will feel comfortable doing it all over! More advanced forms of hydrotherapy, which can have significant effects on the circulation, are described in the chapter on exercise.

Epsom salts are known for their positive effects on the circulation, especially when used as a rub in the shower. Take a small handful of the salts and add some water to make them stick together. Then slowly rub the mixture into the skin, starting with the legs before moving onto the arms and the back, chest and abdomen. After applying the salt, take a brisk shower, rubbing the skin to stimulate the circulation even further. Then wrap up warmly and relax for at least one hour.

Skin brushing is often used to help stimulate the circulation – before a bath or shower (dry brushing) or just afterwards before you dry yourself (wet brushing). Use a loofah and brush gently upwards in a circular motion. You should see a reddening of the skin as the circulation is stimulated.

If you suffer from chilblains or cold hands and feet, try cold water treading. Prepare two bowls, one with hot water, the other with cold. Place your feet in the hot bowl for three minutes and then in the cold bowl for one. Repeat this three to five times, finishing with the cold bowl. Then briskly rub your feet dry with a towel. After this, exercise your toes by flexing them up and down. A walk barefoot in the garden on a frosty morning will produce a similar effect.

If you live near the sea, one of the oldest methods of stimulating the circulation in the feet and legs is simply to walk in the sea. This can have an added beneficial effect for people who suffer from fluid retention as salt water has an osmotic effect and will draw water from the body. The benefits of sea-bathing are described in the chapter on exercise.

Looking after your heart and circulatory system is probably one of the most important things you can do for your health as all the body's systems rely on the heart for their function and well-being. You will be surprised at just how much benefit you can derive from applying some of the suggestions given in this chapter and just how good you will soon feel.

9

How do I care for my skin and hair?

Beauty is, as they say, only skin deep, but that is not much consolation if we feel that we are not looking our best. However much we try not to, we form a large part of our first impression of others by looking at them. When we look at ourselves, what we see reflects not only our health, but also what we think of ourselves, and sends a message to those around us. So, even if we haven't got the face of a supermodel, we owe it to ourselves and to our self-esteem to look – and feel – as fabulous as possible.

Size, and to some degree shape, can be improved by the dietary and exercise measures we referred to in earlier chapters, but the skin and hair need some specific attention to be in tip-top condition.

The skin is the largest organ of the body, covering a surface area of up to 2 square metres (2.5 square yards). It is made up of two layers – the epidermis (the outer layer) and the dermis (the lower layer). The dermis contains the blood and lymph vessels, nerves, nerve endings and hair follicles. Under this is the subcutaneous fatty tissue, which stores most of the body's fat. The epidermis consists of millions of tiny cells that need to be continually fed and nourished to a healthy diet.

When paying attention to our external health and appearance, it is necessary to look inwards, as the internal health of the body will always be reflected on the outside. The composition of the diet is obviously of paramount importance and drinking plenty of water plays a vital part in our daily regime as this affects the quality of the collagen that is laid down in the skin, giving it its elasticity and preventing wrinkles. Glucosamine, an amino acid preparation available from chemists and health food shops, helps to improve the quality of the collagen here, as well as in the tendons and cartilages. The influence of diet on the body and skin is far more effective than any creams or ointment that may be applied externally. This is discussed further in the chapter on eating and drinking healthily. Foods such as pork products, citrus fruits, coffee, tea, alcohol and chocolate are usually the worst culprits in stopping us having the best skin we can.

We should also consider what needs to be taken our of the body. When Dr Vogel and I formulated the Detox Box, a detoxification programme designed to 'spring clean' the body by cleansing the liver, kidneys and so on (see Chapter 1), we often observed the terrific benefit that this treatment had on the skin. A similar effect is also noted after several days of fasting – not only the skin but also the hair and nails benefit. Also of benefit is taking 20 drops of Echinaforce (available from chemists and health food shops), twice a day and using an oil of evening primrose formula. I have formulated such a preparation – called Formula PE – from the company SHP, which is excellent for the skin; it contains royal jelly, cod liver oil powder, vitamin E acetate and evening primrose oil.

You may be surprised to learn that a major factor that can contribute to skin defects is constipation. To help with this, I would recommend taking half a teaspoonful of Dr Vogel's Linoforce, twice a day. This can be obtained from chemists and health food shops. Drinking herbal teas can often bring relief. Nutrition is of paramount importance in dealing with constipation.

Is it, though, possible to hold back the years by looking after our skin and using expensive cosmetics and beauty products? Many pharmacies seem to believe so as they incorporate beauty departments selling a wide range of products by well-known multi-national cosmetic companies as well as stocking medically based products for severe skin problems.

I am often amazed at the opportunities that people take to plaster their faces with products more reminiscent of wall filla than anything else, in an effort to improve themselves. My grandmother, who at the age of ninety-eight still possessed a beautiful skin and a good head of hair, did nothing – other than eating well – to care for her own skin when she was younger, although she recalled that her mother used to smear the pillows with special creams that she had formulated herself to help protect the family's skin. Later on, my grandmother recommended the use of herbal remedies and creams in an effort to maintain a fit and youthful appearance.

Much wisdom and common sense lay in our grandmothers' beauty routines. Their creams and ointments contained marshmallow, colts foot, calendula, sage, St Johns wort, marigold, horsetail, horse chestnut and witch hazel, all of which were used in a variety of different creams. These lotions and potions were applied externally to the skin in an effort to maintain its condition and elasticity.

It is very important to use a regular skin care regime to provide protection against the wind, sunlight, a dry atmosphere, pollution and city grime. It is also necessary for all individuals to ascertain whether their skin is dry, greasy or normal, as lotions, creams and beauty products are formulated specifically for each of these skin types. In addition, recklessly plastering tons of make-up onto the skin can result in irreversible damage. The skin needs to breathe, to be able to assimilate substances such as aromatherapy oils and the ingredients of ointments on its surface, and it is very important that it is regularly cleansed so it can do so. When a good cleanser is used, it is amazing to see the amount of dirt and grime that can be wiped from the skin's surface.

A good skin-care programme should incorporate the use of a cleanser morning and night, followed with a day cream, as well as a night cream to nourish. In addition, be careful when selecting make-up. It is advisable to ensure that the beauty products chosen contain natural ingredients, as for example, do those of the Sans Soucis range, available from the company SHP.

I am constantly asked how Gloria maintains her beautiful complexion. Gloria applies all the principles we have mentioned, paying close attention to what she puts into her body, so that her external appearance radiates health. Whatever she does with regard to cosmetics and make-up only enhances her attractiveness, and these products take only second place to her sensible healthy eating and drinking habits. In addition, Gloria also uses specific remedies such as we describe below to help to maintain the condition of her skin and nails.

As well as adopting these basic principles, we can do more specific things. Hydrotherapy, described in the chapter on exercise, can improve the skin, either directly, or indirectly by stimulating the abdominal organs, alleviating such conditions as dandruff, blackheads and itchy skin. Some suggestions on bath additives are also given in that chapter.

Sometimes it is beneficial to use additional treatment for any unwanted wrinkles. When studying acupuncture, I was most intrigued to learn of 'cosmetic acupuncture' which was demonstrated to me by a colleague in Amsterdam, a highly respected doctor. I was fascinated to learn how this treatment, which tones the skin and increases its elasticity, could be employed in helping to maintain a fabulous skin and complexion, and how this method managed to capitalise on the skin's natural beauty. We successfully worked together on the problems of crows feet, wrinkles, birthmarks and scars left by burns.

By using acupuncture points, as well as laser treatment if necessary, we have developed a very special treatment called the hot room treatment, now carried out by many beauticians. This involves first cleansing, followed by the application of a herbal cream, using hot towels to enable the skin to absorb the cream. Once the cream has been absorbed, acupuncture treatment follows. Once finished, the hot treatment is repeated once more. Laser treatment is then used specifically for crows feet, wrinkles and so on, and then another hot room treatment is given. Normal make-up can then be applied. The before-and-after effects of this treatment are astounding. Women find that their skin is softer and more pliable and that their complexion simply glows with health and beauty.

This treatment can be followed by electro-magnetic light therapy, described in an earlier chapter, which can be used to repair any damage to the skin by improving the quality of the collagen, especially where there may be scarring.

I have found, that together with a natural form of HRT – phytogen (see the chapter on the menopause) – using the remedy Skin Factors from the American company Michaels, which can be obtained from chemists and health food stores, can be of great advantage when extra care and repair of the skin is necessary. Skin Factors is a combination of vitamin A, vitamin E, nicotinamide, zinc, essential fatty acids, red clover, dandelion root and burdock root.

So paying attention and taking extra care of our skin, as well as following the specialist advice of beauticians can result in being able to hold back the years.

At my clinic I see a great number of patients of all ages with skin problems. They want to know the causes, and, in particular, they often enquire why acne is such a common problem. We tend to think of acne as a problem affecting only teenagers, but it is certainly the most common of all skin problems. Very few people are blessed with regular sebaceous glands, hormones, diet and so on further affecting how they work. There are many different types of acne, acne vulgaris being the type mostly affecting young people, but acne rosacea is a frequent problem for the over-fifties.

Acne has its origin in the pores of the skin. Glands in the skin, known as sebaceous glands, produce sebum, a mixture of oil and wax, which lubricates the skin and prevents the loss of moisture. Sebaceous glands are found in the highest concentrations on the face, and, to a lesser extent on the back, chest and shoulders, so it is these areas that acne affects most.

Acne is most common at puberty because certain hormones stimulate changes in the skin that can lead to acne. The male sex hormone testosterone is the major hormonal factor. Although men have a higher level of testosterone than women, there is during puberty an increase of testosterone in both sexes, making girls just as susceptible to acne.

Although acne is considered to be a male hormone-dependent condition, excessive secretion of male hormones is not necessarily the cause, since there is a poor correlation between the blood level of testosterone and the severity of the disease. What appears to be more important is that the skin of patients with acne shows a greater activity of the cnzyme 5-alpha-reductase, which converts testosterone to a more potent form (dihydrotestosterone).

Testosterone causes the sebaceous glands to enlarge and produce more sebum. In addition, the cells that line the skin pores produce more keratin. The combination of an increased secretion of sebum and of keratin can lead to blockage of the pore and the formation of a blackhead. With the pores blocked, bacteria can overgrow and release enzymes that break down the sebum and promote inflammation. This forms what is known as a white head or pimple.

A healthy diet rich in natural whole foods such as vegetables, fruits, whole grains and beans is the finest recommendation for improving acne. All refined and/or concentrated sugars must be eliminated. Foods containing *trans*-fatty acids such as milk, milk products, margarine, shortening and other synthetically hydrogenated vegetable oils, as well as fried foods, must also be avoided. Chocolate is banned on two counts as it is high in both sugar and fats. Milk should be avoided not only because it contains *trans*-fatty acids, but also because it may contain trace levels of hormones. Finally, foods high in iodised salt should be eliminated as some people are quite sensitive to the iodine, a known inducer of acne.

In addition, a number of general measures can be taken. If possible, avoid medications that may cause acne, for example:

- anabolic steroids such as testosterone
- corticosteroids
- oral contraceptives
- progesterone

Try to:

- not take drugs containing bromides or iodides
- avoid exposure to oils and greases
- not use greasy creams in cosmetics
- wash pillowcases regularly in chemical-free detergents – that is ones with no added colours or fragrances
- remove excess sebum and oil from the face by washing thoroughly twice daily (more if necessary)

Very often, however, topical treatments (those applied to the skin) need to be used as well.

Some general guidelines are appropriate when using topical preparations for the treatment of acne regardless of whether they are synthetic or natural. First of all, make sure that the skin is clean and dry. Start treatment slowly to determine the skin's tolerance by applying small amounts to small areas of the affected skin. Skin irritation caused by topical treatments for acne is quite common, even in the weaker over-the-counter preparations. If topical medication results in a rash or irritation, discontinue its use. If the rash does not go away, consult a doctor.

Benzoyl peroxide is by far the most popular topical treatment for mild-to-moderate acne. It is available over the counter without prescription (as Oxy 5, Oxy 10, Clearasil, Benoxyl, etc.). Although the exact action of benzoyl peroxide is not known, it is thought to work as a skin antiseptic to suppress the growth of the bacteria. It is most useful for superficial pimples that are inflamed. In order to be effective, benzoyl peroxide preparations must be applied on a daily basis. The primary side-effects of benzoyl peroxide preparations are that they have a tendency to dry out the skin and/or cause redness and peeling. They can also cause a burning or stinging sensation when applied, and some people develop an allergic rash.

Preparations of the antibiotics tetracycline (Topicycline), erythromycin (A/T/S, Erycette, EryDerm, etc.), and clindamycin (Cleocin T) are used to keep the bacteria under control in the treatment of mild-to-moderate acne. They are available only on prescription. If applied on a regular basis, they can prevent pimple formation. It usually takes three or four weeks of treatment in order to produce a significant improvement. Topical antibiotic preparations can cause skin dryness, tenderness, itching, redness and burning sensations. Some people can develop an allergic rash, and in rare instances, diarrhoea may occur.

Tetracycline has become the 'drug of choice' for most dermatologists in the treatment of acne as it is generally thought to have fewer side effects and yield better results than other antibiotics. When tetracycline cannot be used – with intolerance, for example – erythromycin is used. Similar to the topical antiseptics, tetracycline improves acne by preventing the overgrowth of bacteria in the skin pores. Tetracycline is most effective for the more superficial form of acne affecting the face.

The most common side-effect of tetracycline is the overgrowth of *Candida albicans* and other yeasts in the gastrointestinal and genitourinary tracts. This can result in the appearance of symptoms attributed to systemic candidiasis as well as yeast infections of the mouth, intestinal tract, rectum and/or vagina. Because of this, tetracycline is often prescribed in combination with an antifungal agent (amphotericin B) to prevent yeast overgrowth.

Additional side-effects are the same as for other antibiotics and include allergic reactions, nausea, diarrhoea, vomiting, loss of appetite and colitis. In rare instances, tetracycline can lead to anaemia and low white blood cell and platelet levels.

Retin-A (tretinoin) is a synthetic form of vitamin A that is used in the topical treatment of moderate-to-severe acne and is available only on prescription. It is a harsh medicine that is very difficult to work with. It may also cause an initial worsening of the condition and often takes up to twelve weeks before improvement is obvious. Once an improvement has been seen, a maintenance regime with less frequent applications can be established.

The major side-effects with Retin-A are dry skin and skin irritation. In fact, these side-effects can rarely be avoided. Symptoms can often be quite severe (chemically burning the skin) and require discontinuation of the medication. For this reason, it is best to follow the doctor's recommendation of carefully introducing Retin-A by starting at the lowest concentration possible. Applying more Retin-A than needed does not produce any better a clinical response and will most probably cause marked redness, peeling or severe skin damage.

Isotretinoin is another synthetic derivative of vitamin A, but unlike Retin-A, isotretinoin, or Accutane, is used internally. Because of its high rate of toxicity, Accutane is reserved for the treatment of severe acne that has not responded to other conventional medicines. Accutane should not be used to treat mild-to-moderate acne. Its primary action in the treatment of severe acne is to inhibit the formation of sebum. Accutane must usually be used continuously for five or six months before results are apparent. Like Retin-A, Accutane may cause an initial worsening of the condition.

It is extremely important that individuals taking Accutane be closely monitored by their physician and follow his or her dosage recommendations explicitly. Premenopausal women taking Accutane must use two effective forms of birth control. In virtually every patient, Accutane will cause dryness of the nose and mouth, chapped lips, dry skin and itching, peeling of the palms of the hands and soles of the feet, and elevations of blood cholesterol and triglyceride levels, important in those with heart disease. Women will usually experience vaginal dryness and menstrual changes. Other side-effects, although less common, include allergic reactions, decreased libido, liver damage, thinning of the hair, muscular and joint aches and abnormal bone development.

To try to avoid as many as possible of the potentially aggressive effects of such treatments, Dr Michael Murray, a doctor well known in the USA for his television appearances, and I have worked together on a product called Derma-Clear. This product contains key nutrients for the skin, including vitamins A, C, B3, B5, B6 and B12, minerals, the enzyme bromelain, thymus extract and burdock root extract, all in a base of raw epidermis tissue. When taken at a dose of one capsule, twice a day, this preparation is very effective in clearing many skin ailments. A complete programme of products is available in the Derma-Clear range, from Enzyme Therapy, and a regime incorporating these preparations can be very successful in keeping many skin problems under control. These all-natural products contain no sugar, salt, dairy products, wheat, colouring or flavouring and no irritating fragrances or detergents; they cause no harmful side-effects.

Enzymatic Therapy's Derma-Clear Acne Treatment Programme is guaranteed to be one of the safest and most effective ways to treat and prevent acne. The complete skin care programme includes a soap, cleanser and cream. The cream contains among other things, zinc, sage, hawthorn and chamomile extracts and vitamin E.

One to three times daily, cleanse the skin thoroughly and cover the entire affected area with a thin layer of cream. Because excessive drying of the skin may occur, start with one application daily, and then gradually increase this to two or three times daily if needed or as directed by a doctor. If bothersome dryness or peeling occurs, reduce application to once a day or every other day.

Derma-Clear Acne Treatment Soap contains aloe vera (a natural moisturiser), herbal extracts and sulphur (which supports the body's control of bacteria); it is completely fragrance free. Gently wash your face one to three times daily, leaving the soap on your face for several minutes, then rinse it and pat it dry. If drying or peeling occurs, reduce application to once a day or every other day.

Derma Clear Acne Treatment Cleanser can be used as an alternative to this. It is a natural, hypoallergenic formula containing herbal extracts. Apply the cleanser to your hands or face. Gently wash your face with the cleanser one to three times daily, leaving the cleanser on for several minutes before rinsing and patting dry. If dryness or peeling occurs, reduce the application to once a day or every other day.

So now your skin is looking beautiful and you are beginning to feel fabulous – but what about your hair? Hair is often described as a woman's crowning glory and I feel very sorry for patients who tell me that they are losing their hair or that their hair is thinning. One has to acknowledge that, during the menopause, when deficiencies occur, the hair can become thinner, but it *is* possible to do something about this particular problem.

Hair loss – not the medical condition alopecia that arises for no apparent reason – but hair thinning as a result of not living healthily, is one of the most common complaints of female patients. More and more often, I hear from women that their doctors dismiss the problem of hair loss, saying that it is nothing to worry about. However, if we look more deeply into the situation, we have to realise that we lose between forty and one hundred hairs a day, so it is necessary to encourage new growth all the time.

Between 100,000 and 350,000 hair follicles occupy the human scalp, but not all of these hairs undergo cyclical phases of growth and rest. During the growth (anagen) phase, there is an active genetic expression of protein synthesis. As the hair matures, it enters a resting stage, before the hair bulb migrates outward and is eventually shed. It is during this migratory phase that the stage is set for a new hair to fill the remaining papilla after the original hair has been lost. Age, pathology and a wide variety of nutritional and hormonal factors influence the duration of the hair cycle. Generally speaking, hair loss is a normal part of ageing. By the age of forty or so, the rate of hair growth slows down, so new hairs are not replaced as quickly as old ones are lost. Both men and women suffer from age-related hair loss, but the problem is more apparent in men because of the effects of androgens.

In my experience there are several common causes of hair loss in women, for example medications, nutritional deficiencies, hypothyroidism and excess androgens.

A long list of drugs can cause hair loss. Although all of the drugs listed in the table below are capable of causing hair loss, it should not be assumed that simply because a woman is complaining of hair loss and is taking one of these drugs, that drug is the single cause of her hair loss. For some drugs, of course, most notably chemotherapeutic agents such as fluorouracil, these are obviously the cause.

Classes of drugs that can cause hair loss

Class	Examples
Non-steroidal anti-inflammatory drugs (NSAIDS)	Ibruprofen, indomethacin, naproxen
Antibiotics	Gentamycin, chloramphenicol
Anticoagulants	Coumarins, heparin
Antidepressants	Prozac, desipramine, lithium
Antiepileptics	Valproic acid, dilantin
Cardiovascular drugs	ACE inhibitors, beta-blockers
Chemotherapy drugs	Adriamycin, vincristine, etoposide
Endocrine drugs	Bromocriptine, clomid, danazol
Gout medications	Colchicine, allopurinol
Lipid-lowering drugs	Gemfibrozil, fenofibrate
Ulcer medications	Tagamet, zantac

A deficiency of any of a number of nutrients can lead to significant hair loss. Zinc, vitamin A, essential fatty acids and iron are the nutrients that I consider first and foremost. I examine a patient's nails for the characteristic white lines that indicate poor wound healing of the nail bed (after even the most minor of trauma) as a result of a low zinc level. I examine the back of the arms for hyperkeratosis, a common sign of vitamin A deficiency, and the elbows and general health looking for the dry skin associated with essential fatty acid deficiency. In my experience women with noticeable hair loss will typically be suffering from deficiencies of all these nutrients.

The treatment of hair loss in nutritional deficiency is straightforward: increase the dietary intake of these nutrients and supplement appropriately. In some cases, however, there may be an absorption problem. If the diet contains all the necessary nutrients and there are still problems, the digestive system could be at fault, possibly because of a lack of digestive enzymes. My general recommendation for women with hair loss that I think is related to nutritional status is to take a high-potency multiple vitamin and mineral formula that contains iron, along with one tablespoon of flaxseed oil per day.

I have also been very encouraged by the results obtained using formulae such as Hair and Skin Nutrition – available as tablets and capsules from chemists and health food shops – and by findings with regard to the use of Nutri-Hair. Hair and Skin Nutrition provides a variety of nutrients that the body uses to maintain radiant skin and vibrant hair. Vitamin A and zinc must be included in the diet for skin texture, integrity and moisture. Essential fatty acids support the body oils that keep the skin and scalp in good condition. Other nutrients in Hair and Skin Nutrition must also be present for liver function. The preparation contains in addition a wide range of other vitamins, zinc, lecithin and inositol. The chapter on healthy eating will give you more information on these nutrients.

Nutri-Hair has been formulated to provide certain essential nutrients to help maximise hair growth in women, especially those who have a reduced hair volume compared with that of several years ago or who have recently noticed hair-shedding as seen by more hairs in the brush or comb, or lost when shampooing. Research has shown that a section of the female population, particularly those between 18 and 55, have increased hair-shedding and that there is a strong correlation between this hair loss and low iron stores. Nutri-Hair provides an effective level of iron to correct any dietary deficiency, as well as a high level of the amino acid L-lysine, which plays an important role in the absorption and utilisation of iron. Both of these substances are believed to be present at sub-optimal levels in many people's diets, particularly those who eat little red meat, and in women still menstruating, the low iron intake is obviously compounded by the monthly loss of blood. You can also increase your iron intake by eating plenty of endives or spinach, or by soaking four dried pears in a sweet red port wine overnight. Alternatively, a beaten raw egg in grape juice or red port wine is very beneficial. Taking vitamin C, for example as fruit juice, with an iron supplement helps to increase its absorption.

When Nutri-Hair is taken at the recommended daily dose, there will be a period of at least 12 weeks, more commonly 16, before excessive hair-shedding is reduced. The hair volume will then start to increase, but it takes several months for the hair to grow to a length that contributes to hair volume.

Nutri-Hair can also be used as a high-potency iron supplement for those who consume a diet low in red meat. One tablet, three times a day for the first three months, should be taken as a food supplement. Thereafter, for maintenance purposes one tablet daily can be taken. However, for those who have heavy periods or who eat little or no red meat, two tablets may be required.

Nutri-Hair should not be taken by those taking oral antibiotics, and no other iron-containing supplements should be taken whilst taking it. It should not be taken within two hours of taking any medication, including indigestion remedies.

A small proportion of people may experience some minor digestive disturbances because of the iron contained in Nutri-Hair. This generally disappears, but if it persists, reduce the intake by one tablet.

The condition of the nails often reflects that of the hair and skin, but a couple of supplements may specifically help if you have poor, brittle or weak nails. Dr Vogel's preparation, Urticalcin, available from health food stores and some chemists, often does a wonderful job in improving nail growth. Should there be any fungal problems affecting the growth and condition of the nails, I would recommend using the Edel Propolis Nail Formula, which you can buy in health food shops. I prescribe this preparation on almost a daily basis, and it is of terrific help in eradicating numerous nail problems.

So we can see that becoming the new you that is often advocated and eloquently described in many books and magazines doesn't need to be an arduous and laborious undertaking. Underlying it is just common sense, first and foremost in adhering to a healthy diet and simply cutting out foods that affect the skin negatively. Take positive action by following a detoxification regime, with an occasional fast, getting a good night's sleep, cutting out the foods that adversely affect your skin and using naturally based skin care products, and you will soon see excellent results.

10

How do I cope with the menopause?

Of all the phone-ins that Jan and I have run both on television and on the radio, the biggest reaction by far has come from women with questions about the menopause, or as my mum used to say, 'That Time in Life' for 'The Change'. Even though this is the topic most talked about by women, a recent survey carried out for Lily's women's health and educational television programme showed that an overwhelming majority knew little or nothing about the long-term health risks, even though they could expect to live nearly half of their lives after the menopause.

Almost half of the sample taken did not know what causes the menopause, what happens to the body when the oestrogen level falls as a result or what medical conditions are linked to this relative oestrogen deficiency.

Take heart disease, for example. In Britain alone, every hour nine women die from heart-related problems – that's 80,000 women per year – the vast majority of whom are past the menopause.

Traditionally, until this latest research, heart disease was thought to be a man's problem and women worked hard to make sure that 'their man' did not have a heart attack. Now this is the biggest killer of women. Much, however, can be done to prevent heart disease, as the chapter on looking after your heart and circulation describes.

In addition, one in three women over the age of fifty is at risk of breaking a bone because they have osteoporosis, another condition common after the menopause. This, too, is such an important topic that we have given it a chapter all of its own.

So what is the menopause? It has been suggested by some to be an evolutionary adaptation designed to stop women becoming pregnant in their later years when children could be more hazardous. Others say that we are just living longer so are experiencing more health problems related to this. Whatever the reason, at the time of the menopause, the body's oestrogen level falls. The average British woman experiences the menopause at the age of about forty-eight to fifty, although about 110,000 women annually are affected at a much earlier age and have to learn early to adapt their lifestyle to cope with any symptoms that may arise, and some do not reach the menopause until their mid-to-late fifties.

Nature appears to have intended that the menopause be a gradual process attained by a gradual reduction in the amount of oestrogen produced by the ovaries in the run-up to releasing an egg each month. The oestrogen prepares the uterus in case the egg is fertilised and implants. After the egg has been released, progesterone is produced instead, although some oestrogen remains. If pregnancy does not occur, the levels of both hormones fall and the woman's period begins.

As the function of the ovaries tails off, ovulation becomes irregular and the body's overall oestrogen level drops, the pituitary gland sends signals to the adrenal and other glands to increase their oestrogen output. The oestrogen that is lost from the ovaries is then partially replaced from these sources. It has been suggested that the best menopausal body is one that is a little plump, because the fat cells can convert hormones called androgens into oestrogens and offset the natural fall in these. The level of oestrogen secretion by the adrenals increases naturally in both sexes and, when this back-up supply of oestrogen is working properly, the menopause should occur with few or no side-effects. Indeed, Chinese medicine holds that the menstrual flow should cease without any symptoms at around the age of fifty-six – the later the better since menstruation is considered to be an internal cleansing process. The Chinese actually explain and treat the menopause as a blood deficiency problem. A woman's ability to produce abundant blood declines with age and the process of regularly filling the uterus places a burden upon her kidneys.

Many women in the UK do, however, experience symptoms, depending on the rate at which the oestrogen level falls. A slow decline allows the body to cope more easily, whereas a rapid fall, especially if the woman is stressed, allows little time for adaptation. Although support should be given, the menopause is not, as a lot of people view it, a major illness but a time of change and transition during which a woman's body sheds its child-bearing potential through a lowering of hormone levels.

The menopause may start for many reasons. First, and most commonly, a woman's ovaries may no longer be producing eggs, or she may have ceased to produce the hormones oestrogen and progesterone. The menopause may also arise as a result of chemotherapy or radiotherapy treatment, from damage caused to the ovaries, or as the result of an autoimmune condition. Some women actually continue with their daily lives unaware that they are going through this change, but up to 75 per cent suffer unpleasant symptoms. Despite this, some women are pleased that they have reached the end of their menstruation, as this means that they will no longer have to experience the unpleasant monthly symptoms that are often associated with this.

For most women, the symptoms of the menopause last for two or three years, but others may suffer for as many as five years and their life can become intolerable – hardly a recipe for feeling fabulous.

One of the main symptoms may be heavy menstrual bleeding, which can be frightening and often debilitating for many women, leading to such conditions as iron deficiency anaemia. The chapter on healthy eating suggests how a woman can boost her iron intake.

The second well-known set of symptoms includes hot flushes

and night sweats as the blood vessels dilate. A hot flush is described as a red flare-up of the skin rising up over the face, causing a great deal of discomfort and irritation. Although these occur to a greater or lesser extent in the majority of women, there are some parts of the world, such as Japan, where this problem is virtually unknown, in this case because of a diet rich in phyto-oestrogens, which we discuss in greater detail later on.

Hot flushes are often said to be all in a woman's mind, but I find that the herb Salvia (sage) can be of tremendous assistance in easing the frequency and intensity of hot flushes, and I would specifically advise fifteen drops of Dr Vogel's preparation, Menosan, twice a day. In addition, the remedy Female Essence, a flower essence, available from health food shops, can also be of benefit.

Increasing your exercise level can actually help to reduce the hot flushes, as well as strengthen your bones. According to research, just three and a half hours per week is all that is needed to stave off flushes. Swedish scientists have shown that the brain centre responsible for hot flushes, the hypothalamus, could be reset to normal during exercise. The positive effect of increasing the level of endorphins – the body's natural painkillers – during and after exercise has a balancing action on this key brain centre, helping to normalise the nervous system and stabilise the blood vessels, and thus effectively reducing the severity of the flushing. In time – usually after the first year or so of menopause – the flushing usually subsides.

Difficulty sleeping (which is dealt with in another chapter), bladder problems, loss of skin sensitivity, irregular heart beats and a lower ability to concentrate may also occur at this time. Fatigue and weight gain may occur; for help with the latter, see the chapter on how to control your weight.

Vaginal discharge can be controlled by the homeopathic remedy sepia, whereas the herb spilanthes is used to treat thrush and vaginal infections. Urinary infection often responds to solid age complex.

Another problem area is that of vaginal dryness, leading to painful sexual intercourse. This may add to any relationship problems that the menopause may create. The menopause can be an unsettling and anxious time for many women, and during it they may suffer from a lack of confidence and self-esteem. This can lead to discord within personal relationships and even cause quite a lot of friction with the opposite sex, resulting in difficulties arising within a sexual relationship. When a woman experiences a drop in her libido during the menopause, some partners are understanding, others are not, which makes it more difficult to tackle this tricky area.

Other factors beside hormones may influence how much discomfort the menopausal changes will generate. For example, there is evidence that if you remain sexually active, you will have fewer vaginal problems than if you are celibate or have only occasional sex. Regular sexual activity with your partner seems to increase the amount of lubrication and the ease with which you become lubricated during sexual excitement. It is quite reassuring that medical opinion tells us to remain sexually active as this may help not only to reduce the risk of vaginal problems, but also to enhance our sex life, although sexual activity should not be prescribed as some sort of medication.

The positive benefits of sexual activity are not, however, lost forever after a period of abstinence. As long as intercourse is resumed gradually and carefully, injury to the vaginal tissues can be avoided. After a few weeks of regular sexual activity, lubrication and elasticity should increase. Slow love-making is ideal in attempting to remedy the problem of vaginal dryness or pain during sex because it allows more time for natural lubrication before penetration.

A very good aid for the problem of vaginal dryness is the preparation KY jelly. There are several new and very good creams on the market that can also be of help; Replens, obtainable from chemists shops, is actually one of the best products to use, and should there be an underlying problem – for example an infection with Candida or bacteria – contributing to the difficulties, the excellent product Candida Formula from Enzymatic Therapy can be very helpful.

It is also necessary to be careful when washing with bath foams, or perfumed soaps and bath products. Underwear should preferably be natural cotton, and tight-fitting, nylon underwear should be avoided. Dabbing the affected area of irritation with diluted Molkosan – a milk whey product – can also alleviate chronic irritation. (Molkosan is available from Bioforce.)

A deterioration in the relationship with a partner can combine with the mood swings commonly seen at this time, leading to depression, for which Prozac is often prescribed.

My friend Dr Michael Murray, the well-known American

physician, writes that there are a number of psychological therapies that can be quite useful in helping to eliminate depression. The therapy that I feel has the most merit and support in medical literature is cognitive therapy. This has been shown to be equally as effective as antidepressant drugs in treating moderate depression. However, while there is a high rate of relapse of depression when drugs are used, the relapse rate with cognitive therapy is much lower. People taking drugs for depression tend to have to stay on them for the rest of their lives, but this is not the case with cognitive therapy because the patient is taught new skills to deal with depression.

Psychologists and other mental health specialists trained in cognitive therapy seek to change the way in which a depressed person consciously thinks about failure, defeat, loss and helplessness. Cognitive therapists employ five basic tactics. First they help patients to recognise the negative thoughts that flit through their consciousness at the times when they feel worst. The second tactic is disputing the negative thoughts by focusing on contrary evidence. The third tactic is teaching the patient a different explanation to dispute the negative automatic thoughts. Fourth, the treatment involves methods of avoiding rumination (the constant churning of a thought in one's mind) by helping patients better to control their thoughts. The final tactic is questioning depression-causing negative thoughts and beliefs, and replacing them with empowering positive thoughts and beliefs.

Cognitive therapy does not involve the long, drawn-out process of psychoanalysis. It is a solution-orientated psychotherapy designed to help the patient learn skills to improve the quality of his or her life. If your thought processes are in need of a little re-wiring, consult a mental health specialist who practises cognitive therapy.

Depression may also have an organic or physiological cause, such as pain from for example osteoporosis, or the taking of prescription drugs. It is essential to eliminate easily reversible organic causes of depression before taking an antidepressant drug. Common drugs associated with causing depression include corticosteroids, beta-blockers and other antihypertensive medications. In addition, substances not often considered to be drugs, such as oral contraceptives, alcohol, caffeine and cigarettes, can cause depression by disrupting the normal balance between brain neurotransmitters. For most medical conditions there are natural medicines, without side-effects, that will produce better results than drugs.

Nervous conditions or other hormonal imbalances may disrupt the menstrual cycle, leaving women at risk of bone loss and heart disease as an unwanted knock-on effect. Such conditions must be treated to avoid this.

Given the sometimes dramatic effects of the menopause, and the fact that it may go on for years, is it a good idea to take hormone replacement therapy (HRT) to try to counteract them? Known by some as the 'elixir of youth', HRT, which contains oestrogen and occasionally a progesterone-like substance, has been disregarded by others, resulting in mass confusion all round. Rarely does a month go by without some new twist to the advice given to women with regard to the use of HRT. The use of synthetic oestrogen has been described as the largest uncontrolled clinical trial in history, so it is not surprising that we are ill informed with regard to its effects.

There are definitely some benefits from taking HRT – it will stop hot flushes and counteract urinary tract infections and urinary leakages, and even help to maintain a youthful complexion, and its effect on the bones can be profound. When it comes to severe osteoporosis, HRT may stabilise the situation and even prevent a bone fracture following a minor fall. In such cases, it will obviously be considered as part of treatment, but all too often it is prescribed without good cause for something that is a natural biological change rather than an illness. In addition, the benefits of HRT do not often outweigh the problems that arise as a consequence. First, let's take a look at these, before going on to look at other ways of dealing with the problem.

The side-effects of HRT include:

- an increased risk of cancer of the uterus
- an increased risk of breast cancer
- an increased risk of gallstones and jaundice
- high blood pressure
- an increased risk of stroke or heart attack
- nausea and vomiting
- the symptoms of PMS
- breast tenderness, vaginal bleeding and the aggravation of fibroystic disease of the breast

- depression
- weight gain
- liver disorders
- the enlargements of any pre-existing uterine fibroids
- fluid retention
- blood sugar disturbances
- headaches
- the aggravation of migraine attacks
- irritation of the eyes when wearing contact lenses

Women with the following conditions may find that they are aggravated by taking HRT:

- migraine
- high blood pressure
- heart or kidney disease
- a melanoma
- diabetes
- otosclerosis (a condition leading to deafness)
- multiple sclerosis
- the connective tissue disorder systemic lupus erythematosus
- endometriosis
- uterine fibroids
- circulatory problems
- chronic liver disease with abnormal liver function tests

It is reported that, of all the women who choose HRT, one-third stop taking it within nine months, more than half quitting within a year because of its side-effects.

The number of women approaching me for help for breast cancer nowadays has significantly increased. Drugs designed to treat certain illnesses may cause specific side-effects, including many of the breast cancers that I have seen in the over-fifties. So, if a woman decides to take oestrogen, it will be necessary for her to attend for regular examinations and check-ups – not only for breast cancer but also for cancer of the uterus. The PAP cervical smear, however, is designed only for cervical examinations and will not pick up abnormal tissue in the uterus. Despite this, the tests are necessary and have undoubtedly saved many lives. It is certainly better to be safe than sorry, especially in view of the fact that, in the UK, the death rate for cervical cancer, which used to be quite low, has not dropped despite the 40 million smear tests carried out annually and is indeed now on the increase; so it seems as if, overall, we are more at risk of this condition.

Let us digress for a moment to take a closer look at breast cancer. It is currently estimated that one out of seven women in the USA will develop breast cancer at some time during their lives. More than 150,000 cases are detected and more than 50,000 deaths occur each year in the USA. These statistics are frightening; virtually every American has known someone who has been struck with this deadly illness. The rate of breast cancer is typically five times higher for women in the USA than women in other parts of the world. While a genetic predisposition is an important risk factor, it is in most cases secondary to the more important dietary, lifestyle and environmental factors: in Japan, the rate of breast cancer is about one fifth the rate in the USA, but in second- or third-generation Japanese women living in America who eat the standard American diet, the rate of breast cancer is identical to that of other women living in the USA. The table below provides a list of the factors that have been linked to breast cancer.

Possible causes of breast cancer

Genetic factors

Hormonal factors (increased oestrogen exposure)
Early onset of menstruation
Pregnancy late in life or not at all
Late menopause
Shorter menstrual cycles

Environmental factors
Xeno-oestrogens (synthetic compounds that mimic oestrogen)
Pesticides, herbicides, halogenated compounds, etc.
Lack of sunlight
Power lines, electric blankets, radiation, etc.

Iatrogenic (treatment induced) factors
Oral contraceptives

Hormone replacement therapy
Radiation (diagnostic and therapeutic)
Chemotherapy

Lifestyle factors
Exposure to cigarette smoke
Body weight (the more overweight, the greater the risk)
Exercise level (women who exercise have a reduced rate)
Alcohol and coffee consumption

Dietary factors
Increased saturated fat
Decreased anti-oxidants
Decreased dietary fibre
Decreased alpha-linolenic acid and omega-3-fatty acids
Decreased dietary phyto-oestrogens

It has been suggested that prophylactic mastectomy might be of benefit to those with a family history of the disease. One retrospective study consisted of all women with a family history of breast cancer who underwent bilateral prophylactic mastectomy in the Mayo Clinic between 1960 and 1993, following them up for an average of fourteen years. The women were divided into two groups – high and moderate risk – on the basis of their family history. A control study of the sisters of those in the high-risk group and a mathematic model were used to predict the number of breast cancers in these two groups in the absence of prophylactic mastectomy. It was found that a 90 per cent reduction in the rate of breast cancer occurred in the moderate-risk group after mastectomy.

So given the growing number of women who have a family history of breast cancer, do these results indicate that prophylactic mastectomy should be the primary preventative measure for these women? It is hard to argue against the numbers, but prophylactic mastectomy seems to be a very aggressive preventative measure. Instead, I believe that the focus should be on diet and lifestyle.

Conventional breast cancer prevention is mostly aimed at surveillance, such as mammograms and self-examination, and in some cases drugs, for example tamoxifen, but dietary factors appear to be critical components of the prevention of breast cancer. In fact, it is estimated that dietary intervention could reduce the risk of breast cancer by at least 80 per cent (fairly close to the level produced by prophylactic mastectomy in the study above).

The research in this area is often somewhat unclear because investigators often evaluate dietary factors only in the USA. For example, let's take a look at the research on saturated fats and breast cancer. It is difficult to determine true risk when looking at women in the USA because the lowest percentile for saturated fat intake in the USA often translates to the highest percentile in other countries. To gauge all the dietary risk factors in breast cancer, it is extremely important to examine data from a global perspective. This assessment has been made, and, in my opinion, provides the best evidence of which dietary factors appear to promote breast cancer and which appear to be preventative and causative. The table below lists these factors in descending order of preventing or causing cancer. Clearly, eating a diet primarily composed of preventative agents while avoiding causative agents should be encouraged to prevent breast cancer.

Dietary factors linked to causing breast cancer	Dietary factors linked with preventing breast cancer
Animal products	Fish
Meats	Whole grains
Total fat content	Legumes (pulses)
Saturated fats	Cabbage
Dairy produce	Vegetables
Refined sugar	Nuts
Total number of calories	Fruits
Alcohol	

One of the most interesting aspects of the population study noted above was the tremendous protective effect of fish consumption. Fish, particularly cold water fish such as salmon, mackerel, halibut and herring, are rich sources of the omega-3 fatty acids. This group of oils has shown tremendous anti-cancer effects against breast cancer in experimental studies. In contrast, the omega-6 fatty acids found in most animal products, as well as in common vegetable oils such as corn, safflower and soy, are associated with promoting breast cancer in experimental studies.

In addition to a diet that features fish, supplementing the diet with flaxseed oil appears to offer significant protection against breast cancer, for several different reasons. First of all, flaxseed oil contains nearly twice the amount of omega-3 fatty acids as do fish oils. In one study looking at 121 women with initially localised breast cancer, the lower level of alpha-linolenic acid in the breast tissue, the more the cancer invaded and spread (metastasised) round the body. Since the main cause of death of breast cancer patients is the development of cancer in other tissues, this finding is of extreme importance. The results from this study suggest that supplementing the diet with flaxseed oil (approximately 58 per cent alpha-linolenic acid) may help to prevent cancer, invasion and metastasis.

There have been warnings based on the results of some studies that it is unwise to supplement with flaxseed oil in both prostate and breast cancer. However, it appears that alpha-linolenic acid is an 'innocent bystander' in these reports. In the absence of vegetable sources of alpha-linolenic acid, blood and tissue levels of alpha-linolenic acid reflect meat intake. This is exactly what these studies linking alpha-linolenic acid to breast and prostate cancers have demonstrated – that a higher meat intake increases the risk of prostate and breast cancer. The high level of meat intake in these studies was also associated with an extremely high intake of saturated fats and cholesterol and a very high ratio of omega-6 to omega-3 fatty acids. Such a ratio has been suggested to be an important risk factor in breast cancer.

In addition to containing large amounts of alpha-linolenic acid, flaxseeds and flaxseed oil are also the most abundant sources of lignans. Plant lignans are changed by micro-organisms in the gut into enterolacton and enterodiol, two compounds that are believed to be protective against cancer, particularly breast cancer. These phyto-oestrogens (see later in the chapter) are capable of binding to the oestrogen receptors on the cells and interfering with the cancer-promoting effects of oestrogen on breast tissue. Lignans also help to regulate oestrogen levels by promoting the removal of oestrogen from the body via eliminative pathways. Since exposure to oestrogens is a major risk factor in breast cancer, foods containing lignans and other phyto-oestrogens, such as soy and whole grains, are thought to protect against breast cancer.

Population studies, as well as experimental studies on humans and animals, have demonstrated that lignans exert significant anti-cancer effects. In an animal experiment, flaxseed oil or flaxseed demonstrated a significant reduction in tumour number and size after one or two months.

While soy phyto-oestrogens seem to get all the attention, lignans appear to offer much greater protection. In a recent case-control study of phyto-oestrogens and breast cancer, a high urinary excretion of enterolactone (from lignan metabolism) provided a far greater reduction in breast cancer risk compared with daidzein, a major phyto-oestrogen of soy.

So although we can take some steps to decrease our risk of breast cancer, it still remains a significant side-effect of HRT.

There is some truth in the fact that combining the oestrogen with progesterone eliminates many of the side-effects, but it must be remembered that even the combined form of HRT carries its own list of potential health complications. Progesterone, in the form of synthetic progestins, is known to aggravate pre-existing high blood pressure, diabetes, and liver, heart and kidney disease as well as being responsible for a whole host of other effects such as dangerous blood clots, fluid retention, breast tenderness, jaundice, nausea, insomnia and depression. Many women who are taking a progestin often report that the hormone makes them feel just plain awful. In addition, most women who take a combination of oestrogen and progestin have a return of menstrual bleeding, and this may require periodic biopsies of the uterine lining to screen for cancer.

With all this in mind the obvious question 'Is there an alternative?' arises. As the following story shows, there is certainly a need for one. I recall recently seeing a woman at my clinic who told me how important sex was in her life. Basically, she had enjoyed a regular and satisfying sex life, but after a hysterectomy her sex life changed dramatically. She became very depressed, and although her doctor had recommended HRT, she did not want to try it. Besides the loss of sexual arousal and desire, she was experiencing other problems that led to her becoming even more depressed. Fortunately, upon starting her off on some alternative natural remedies based on vitamins, minerals and trace elements, as well as Women's Formula (a preparation available from chemists to give the libido a boost), she regained much of her former enthusiasm and zest for life.

The obvious place to start, as we have often said in this book, is with our diet. The chapter on eating and drinking healthily will give you an overview of this area. Good foods, a good eating pattern and good digestion can stimulate the regular functioning of the endocrine glands. A thyroid imbalance often occurs at the time of the menopause, leading to a lack of trace elements such as iodine or manganese, so these may need to be supplemented. It is of benefit to add extra vitamin E (800–1200 units daily) and vitamin C (1000–3000 mg daily) to your diet.

Raw and fresh fruits and vegetable juices are important, as are nuts and dried fruits, which help to maintain the body's potassium level, important in controlling the symptoms of arthritis. It is also important to pay close attention to the heart, as this organ can become affected and possibly degenerate during the menopausal years.

Some of the foods in our diet contain oestrogen-like substances, so it seems obvious to use these as a sort of 'natural HRT'. If we can support and control the body's functions naturally, it seems preferable to do so rather then run the risk of using a preparation that may cause side-effects more serious than the initial complaint. With the ever-growing body of evidence indicating that tradition HRT preparations have the potential to cause serious, sometimes life-threatening side-effects, the search for safe, effective natural alternatives is gaining momentum.

Our evolutionary history clearly shows that man's dietary habits have dramatically moved away from a stable intake of vegetables and pulses towards more highly processed and fundamentally nutritionally deficient food. Our gross intake of food and energy calories may have increased, but nutritional quality has taken a definite turn for the worse!

But it should come as no surprise, especially to those who study health and disease from a biological point of view, that nature has, from the start, supplied the answer to the menopause and our growing decline in the quality of female health; we have just turned out backs on it in favour of the newly found 'fruits' of modern living. This natural elixir can be found in the group of vegetables known as legumes. These foods appear to hold the key to buffering the adaptation to the hormonal changes associated with the menopause. Medicine in its wisdom has developed hormones to replace the ones lost over this natural transition, but there is no such thing as a free lunch: you cannot simply replace a natural hormone with an artificial one and hope that everything will run smoothly.

Few natural substances have recently received so much scientific attention as the phyto-oestrogens (literally plant oestrogens). The frenzy of research is currently generating over forty scientific papers each week, and with good reason, as phyto-oestrogens are set to revolutionise the management of the menopause and its related mid-life health problems.

One of the richest sources of biologically active phyto-oestrogens can be found in the red clover plant (*Trifolium pratense*). This plant contains all four of the important isoflavones that have been identified to be the protective components of traditional diets commonly associated with reduced menopausal complications. These observations originated from studies of the dietary habits of Eastern, Mediterranean and Latin American communities. These populations consume on average between 30 and 100 mg of isoflavones per day. They enjoy many health benefits when compared with the typical Western cultures; women in the UK generally eat less than 3 mg of isoflavones daily.

In cultures that eat large amounts of soya, which is naturally high in phyto-oestrogens, certain diseases, for example breast cancer, are noted to be rare. Interestingly, over 80 per cent of women in the UK suffer from hot flushes, compared with fewer than 10 per cent in Japanese populations. Large-scale studies have indicated that the Japanese diet contains large quantities of vegetable protein such as soy – as much as 40–60 g per day. The UK diet on the whole is very low in this type of protein. However, these cultures also have a diet low in animal fats and alcohol, both known risk factors for cancer. Phyto-oestrogens appear to exert their beneficial effects by lowering the oestrogen level as a result of controlling the way in which it is transported in the blood to the tissues.

Out of the vast array of over a thousand isoflavones, four – genistein, daidzein, biochanin A and formononetin – have been identified as having oestrogenic (oestrogen-like) activity. These active compounds are found in a wide range of fruit and vegetables, especially the pulses, which form the bulk of a typical vegetarian diet. Foods such as soy, chick peas, broad beans, lentils, red clover, green split peas and Chinese peas all contain beneficial amounts of isoflavones, but only red clover can boast significant amounts of the four oestrogenically active compounds. Other plants rich in natural oestrogens are celery, fennel, rhubarb, and green and yellow vegetables, especially exotic members of the cabbage and turnip family.

The interest in red clover grew from the observation that sheep grazing on clover in New Zealand suffered a high rate of miscarriage. Further studies demonstrated that the level of phyto-oestrogens in the sheep's body was so great that the uterus was overstimulated and the pregnancy lost. In this unusual case, it must be kept in mind that the animals fed almost exclusively on clover had managed to attain unnaturally high levels in their bodies. The normal human dietary consumption of phyto-oestrogens, even in those populations who traditionally consume large amounts of legumes, could never reach anywhere near the hazardous levels inadvertently ingested by the sheep: where the sheep ate kilograms of clover daily, humans tend to eat leguminous vegetables in milligram quantities.

As a result of this finding, research became intense, and the data has been mounting in favour of supplementing the Western diet with isoflavones derived from red clover. In a very recent study, fifty post-menopausal women were randomly allocated to two treatment groups. The first group took a placebo tablet (one containing no active agent but looking like the real thing), while the second group took a standardised 40 mg red clover extract. Both groups took the tablets for twelve weeks, after which time, unbeknown to them, their tablets were swapped around for fourteen weeks. This meant that the red clover group took the placebo and the placebo group took the red clover extract. This type of clinical trial is referred to as a crossover placebo study. During the study, the women kept symptom diaries, and blood samples were taken at regular intervals to assess the effect of treatment on the blood and its chemicals. At the end of the study, the results showed that low-dose supplementation gave rise to beneficial effects in the red clover group, who excreted more isoflavones in their urine than did the placebo group. Hot flushes were reduced, and there were no adverse effects to report from the blood tests.

Where heart disease is concerned, the interest in supplementing the diet with isoflavones has been great, especially in the light of the increased risk of venous thrombosis associated with traditional HRT. Looking again at populations who have a high isoflavone phyto-oestrogen intake, the incidence of heart disease, particularly in post-menopausal women, is very low. The selling point of HRT is the fact that the oestrogen influences cholesterol metabolism and leads to high levels of HDL ('good' cholesterol) and lower levels of LDL ('bad' cholesterol), as well as reducing the tension in the muscular walls of the arteries and so easing the flow of blood. Clinical studies of isoflavone supplements given to post-menopausal women have demonstrated effects on vascular function similar to those observed with HRT. Dietary isoflavones have been shown to improve cardio-vascular fitness and reduce risk factors such as high cholesterol and hardening of the arteries. Red clover extracts with a standardised isoflavone content therefore offer an attractive alternative to the standard HRT prescription.

Looking towards a nutritional alternative to extracts of red clover, great interest has focused on the staple food soya. It is interesting to note that there is no word in the Japanese language for menopause, which probably reflects the lack of menopausal symptoms reported by the population in general. It is no secret that Japan has one of the lowest incidents of breast cancer in the world, with low incidence of osteoporosis and related fractures following closely on. Hot flushes are also a rare symptom reported by women during the menopause. Much of this can be attributed to their diet, which is rich in soya protein, often up to 40–60 g per day. Contained within this staple diet is a high concentration of phyto-oestrogens.

One of the key issues surrounding the benefit gained from soya phyto-oestrogens is the ratio of genistein to daidzein, which is found to be in the region of 3:2. This can be exploited in therapeutic soya extracts such as that contained in the product Phytogen, an excellent remedy I have recently discovered that can be used as a natural alternative to HRT. The exact same ratio has been standardised in Phytogen, then concentrated by a factor of a hundred and further standardised to contain 13–17 per cent of isoflavones. This highly purified and standardised soya supplement, taken in a dose of one capsule twice a day, delivers the key factors required to effectively tackle menopause symptoms naturally, often within two or three months of starting the programme.

Also contained within Phytogen, which is produced by Enzymatic Therapy, are:

- vitamin E, for cardiovascular function
- flaxseed oil, which is rich in lignins and may be linked to the sex hormones
- gamma-oryzanol from rice bran, which has been studied for its action in lowering the cholesterol level by promoting the excretion of cholesterol in the faeces; it also helps to reduce anxiety
- pumpkin seed oil, which is rich in essential fatty acids and sterols; essential fatty acids are known to be vital for sexual gland function
- saponins, the oestrogenic compounds of soy

As mentioned above, some synthetic HRT preparations also contain progesterone-like substances, which can be of benefit in counteracting menopausal symptoms. The progesterone in the body is quite different from that found in HRT preparations. As natural progesterone cannot be patented by pharmaceutical manufacturers, the shape of the natural progesterone has to be changed to a new form that can be patented and mass-produced. This altered progesterone works to some degree in the human body, but because it is not identical to the natural compound, side-effects soon follow. Thus replacing HRT with natural progesterone, as in Pro-gest and Phytogen, is likely to be of benefit. Sometimes only a little is needed to make a big impact, just like the ripples that move across a pond when we throw a stone into the water.

One of the best publicised HRT alternatives is Mexican yam, its extracts and creams. Contained within the Mexican yam is a chemical, diosgenin, that, with the aid of another chemical, can be converted into progesterone identical to that found in nature. This second chemical does not, however, occur in the body, so the process has to be carried out in a laboratory. Once this reaction has occurred, the final product contains active progesterone and is therefore classified as a hormone-based product, so it can only be prescribed by a doctor. All other Mexican yam products contain unconverted diosgenin rather than active progesterone and can be sold without a prescription, but it must be remembered that the body cannot convert diosgenin into progesterone.

Many women suffering menopausal symptoms will benefit from

taking the preparation Female Balance (obtained from Enzymatic Therapy), in a dose of fifteen drops twice a day. It is also useful if symptoms of premenstrual syndrome are still in evidence. Female Balance contains essential vitamins and minerals – for example, vitamins A, B1, B2, B12, C and E, iron, zinc, folic acid and selenium – which are often deficient at such a time. These are combined with concentrated extracts of herbs that women have depended on for centuries – extracts of Dong Quai, licorice root, black cohosh, chaste berry and milk thistle. Nowadays, black cohosh and *Agnus castus* are often used alone; both are available from chemists and health food shops. The first four of these extracts are also contained in the preparation Fembrol, from Enzymatic Therapy.

The supplement Gynovite Plus, formulated by Dr Guy Abraham for women during and after the menopause and available from Lamberts, contains a number of trace elements, minerals and vitamins. This multivitamin and multimineral supplement has been designed to be used as part of a total dietary programme to help to safeguard the proper nutritional requirements of these women. The product contains twenty-eight ingredients, with a particular emphasis on the minerals essential for helping to maintain optimum health, and it can be taken either alongside HRT or on its own. The formula does not overemphasise calcium since Dr Abraham has found that magnesium is just as essential for bone health, and this mineral is often likely to be deficient if the diet is not well balanced. Adequate magnesium facilitates the absorption of calcium, so less calcium is needed in the supplement.

A variety of other remedies may also be of help. Even simple ones such as Osteoprime and Urticalcin, to boost calcium levels, can be used.

If there are mood swings, such as Jekyll and Hyde tendencies, it will be helpful to use some hormone-balancing remedies such as an evening primrose oil preparation formulated for the menopause.

Where there is depression, a remedy such as Hypericum Complex, from health food shops, which is a natural substitute for Prozac, can be very effective. Depression may also arise from a stagnation of the liver meridian. When the liver is not functioning efficiently, the blood does not flow freely and the liver is unable to perform its cleansing function efficiently. As a result, hormones are not broken down effectively, and depression is the ensuing result. When the energy flow stagnates, a sensation of sluggishness and lethargy is also felt within the body. Liver energy is very important, so it is important to use Milk Thistle Complex, a special remedy formulated by Dr Vogel, and available in health food shops, to help support the function of the liver, taken in a dose of fifteen drops twice a day after meals.

Putting together all we have learnt above, the following recipe for a 'natural' HRT cake may be a welcome addition to the diet during the menopause. Take:

- 4 oz (100 g) of soya flour
- 4 oz (100 g) of wholewheat flour (although wholemeal will do instead)
- 4 oz (100 g) of porridge oats
- 8 oz (200 g) of raisins (or sultanas, cherries or chopped apricots)
- two pieces of stem ginger
- 140 ml (quarter pint) of soya milk. (As this mixture is extremely stiff, you will probably need to add a bit of water as well. The mixture should not be runny, but 'squelchy')
- two tablespoons of malt extract (more if you like)
- 4 oz (100 g) linseeds (mill these in a grinder or food processor if you can)
- 2 oz (50 g) sunflower seeds
- 2 oz (50 g) pumpkin seeds
- 2 oz (50 g) sesame seeds
- half a teaspoon of cinnamon
- half a teaspoon of nutmeg
- half a teaspoon of ground ginger
- 2 oz (50 g) of flaked almonds (optional). (These are not essential because they are expensive and fattening, and make no real difference to the finished cake)

The larger seeds can also be broken up in a food processor, but not too much or the texture of the cake may suffer. The linseeds benefit most from a good grinding and the sesame seeds are obviously too small to need breaking up. Soak the seeds in some of the soya milk for an hour. (You can also add the water if you like.) You can use sweetened soya milk if you prefer and also some syrup from the jar of stem ginger. Honey would probably also give it a bit of a boost. Another handy tip is to mix the flour, soya flour and porridge oats together as this helps to disperse the soya flour evenly. Then mix in the rest of the soya milk, followed by everything else.

The quantity of mixture is enough for two 1lb loaf tins, which should be lined with baking parchment or oiled greaseproof paper. Bake for about an hour at 180°C/350°F/gas mark 4. The cake will go slightly brown on top and will become very firm to the touch. It can be frozen until needed. The daily 'dose' is 4 oz (100 g)

So it can be seen that the natural treatment of menopause-related symptoms is possible, but it is important to locate good-quality products, preferably with standardised doses of the natural extracts. It is unfortunate that many people lose faith in natural medicine simply because the remedy they used was not strong enough or just plainly ineffective. If you choose carefully and understand your needs, your body should respond.

Women play an increasingly active role in modern society, and it is important that the fundamental stresses and strains of life's experiences do not upset or adversely affect the finely tuned harmony within the body. It is important to ensure that, during this challenging part of life, a woman maintains her self-esteem and self-confidence by continuing to keep healthy, happy and looking fabulous. One way to do this is to be in control of your own destiny. As Gloria puts it, no-one will look after your long-term health after the menopause but *you*, so arm yourself with the facts in order that the next time you visit your doctor you will be able to talk about not only the symptoms of your menopause, but also the quality of your long-term life. Take responsibility for your health into your own hands.

It is often said that one of the most creative forces in the world is a menopausal woman with a zest for life, so let that woman be you.

11

How do I stave off osteoporosis?

Osteoporosis is a condition characterised by thinning of all the bones in the body, with a gradual reduction in the bone mass, resulting in weakening of the skeleton. It can have a medical cause, such as thyroid gland malfunction, or occur for no apparent reason. Although it starts at about the age of thirty-five in women and can also occur in men, it becomes much more apparent after the menopause as a result of the falling oestrogen level, which we discussed in the previous chapter. If nothing is done to counteract this, a woman could lose up to 30 per cent or more of her bone mass by the time she is seventy, although it tends to tail off after this.

The rate at which the oestrogen drops determines the rate of bone loss, and this is the most important factor in determining whether a woman will be at risk of breaking a bone.

In the UK, one in three women over the age of fifty are at risk of breaking a bone because of their osteoporosis. In the USA, osteoporosis is a major epidemic, affecting a third of all American women and being responsible for at least a million fractures a year, usually of the hips, ribs or wrists. The medical and social costs of this are estimated to be $6 billion annually, added to which are the personal costs of pain, hospitalisation and immobility. Preventing fractures depends on preserving enough mineral (primarily calcium and phosphorus) in the bone, preventing the loss of the protein matrix on which this is deposited, and ensuring that damaged areas of bone can be adequately repaired.

As Gloria says, it is a sobering thought that most education about osteoporosis is aimed at those over the age of menopause whereas the reality is that young people should also be very conscious about how they lay the foundation for strong healthy bones in their teenage years and early twenties. What you put into your body then determines how dense your bone will be in later life when you reach the menopause.

So how can a woman tell whether she is developing osteoporosis? Unfortunately, no routine testing is available so a problem has to develop before the doctor can arrange further investigation. Such a problem may be bone pain, a badly rounded back (a 'dowager's hump') interfering with breathing, or even a fracture after some minor trauma. Modern methods of diagnosis can, however, detect early changes in bone density before physical signs can be seen.

The reduction in bone strength associated with osteoporosis results from a loss of the collagen framework onto which calcium and other minerals are deposited under the influence of oestrogen. Collagen loss is a normal change associated with the onset of the menopause. Within a couple of years, this loss normally slows down, and the related calcium loss diminishes. The diagnosis of osteoporosis is difficult using conventional X-ray methods as over 35–40 per cent of the bone mineral needs to have been lost in order for it to be detected on X-rays.

Bone densiometry scanning (DXA scanning) has now become the 'gold standard' for the diagnosis and monitoring of bone loss and gain. However, DXA scanning has a drawback; if a low bone density is detected, the only way of finding out how 'aggressively' the bone loss is occurring is to re-scan about eighteen months later. Over this time, a considerable amount of bone mineral may be lost or an inappropriate prescription of HRT and/or bisphosphonate medication may be started.

To determine the 'aggressiveness' of the bone loss, a simple urine test (an Ntx test) can be used to estimate the amount of chemicals lost that relate to bone turnover. When taken alone (without the results of a DXA scan), the Ntx test will give a good idea of the risk of developing osteoporosis within one year. When used in conjunction with DXA, any osteoporosis detected can then be viewed as being active 'aggressive', active or inactive, and the appropriate treatment can be recommended.

When undergoing osteoporosis treatment, the Ntx test can also be used to monitor the response to any treatment (conventional or alternative) that has been given. As the bone loss slows down, so does collagen breakdown, and therefore the level of Ntx falls in the urine. As the bone eventually rebuilds, the DXA scan will show an improvement, but this is not as sensitive to change as the Ntx test and may take eighteen months to two years to show encouraging results, compared with two or three months for the Ntx test. It only takes a 5–8 per cent increase in bone mineral density to greatly reduce the risk of fracture; as we have said above, the risk of a fracture depends more on the rate of bone loss than the absolute extent of the osteoporosis.

The best way to avoid the problems of osteoporosis is to make sure the bone is as strong as possible before the menopause, by adopting a healthy diet and taking weight-bearing exercise. But whatever the state of her skeleton as she enters the menopause, a woman owes it to herself to care for her bones during this time so that she can prevent as much osteoporosis as possible. We need to learn and think about what we do.

Exercise will continue to be important, but it must be weight-bearing, for example tennis or cycling, for it to have an effect. Swimming, although excellent for the heart and for keeping the joints mobile, will not help as much to increase the bone density. You can find some more ideas in the chapter on exercise.

Smoking is very bad for the bones, as well as for the heart, which provides two good reasons to give it up. Drinking too much alcohol has the same effect.

The next step we can take is to change our diet. As Gloria and I have said so many times in this book, the basis of good health is paying attention to what we eat. Obviously, a good balanced diet incorporating lots of fruit and vegetables is vitally important. To make sure that the body is able to make healthy bone, we need also to ensure that we have sufficient protein, calcium and other minerals and vitamins.

As Gloria writes, one of the main problems here is that most of us go on a weight-loss diet at some point in our lives, and as soon as we cut out dairy produce, as we are advised to because of its fat content, we automatically cut out calcium. So we have to learn how to put calcium back into our bodies. Calcium-rich foods include broccoli, beans, spinach and other green vegetables, low-fat yoghurt and cheese, whitebait, certain breads, mineral water, skimmed milk and even tea. Research shows that three or four cups of tea a day will provide up to 16 per cent of our calcium requirements, and current medical research also highlights tea's ability to reduce the risks of high blood pressure and coronary heart disease.

If the bone is of low quality before the menopause starts, dietary support may be required. Taking a moderate dose of calcium (600–800 mg per day) in addition to other nutrients such as magnesium, boron, vitamin D and vitamin K will help. Dr Vogel thought of using stinging nettles, a plant rich in calcium, to make up a specific homeopathic preparation. I have had many positive results from this product, Urticalcin, available from health food shops. It should be taken at a dose of five tablets, twice a day. In the average woman a daily intake of calcium above 200 mg is not likely to provide any additional benefit.

But healthy bones need more than calcium. Vitamin D is necessary to utilise the calcium and phosphorus properly. Magnesium activates the enzymes that help to form new calcium crystals. Vitamin K is involved in the production of osteocalcin, the supporting structure on which calcium crystallises in bone. Studies show that manganese, zinc, strontium, vitamin B6 and C, silicon, copper and boron, often deficient in Western diets, also help to form the connective structures in bone. A balanced combination of these important nutrients, as well as others, can be found in the supplement Osteoprime, available from health food shops. Two tablets should be take twice daily during or after meals, as an addition to the everyday diet. Osteoprime should not be used if you are already taking a coumarin or warfarin anticoagulant as it may alter the action of these medications.

Potassium-rich foods such as potatoes, bananas, dried fruits, cider vinegar and molasses can be eaten in increased amounts. Apples, grapes, pears, leafy green vegetables, spinach, parsley, broccoli, beets, grains, nuts, dried beans and lentils are all very rich in boron. When there is a problem with boron deficiency, Osteoguard, a remedy from Lamberts is beneficial. Boron and magnesium help to guide the deposition of calcium into the bones instead of the soft tissues of the body. It is this relationship between these two minerals that has led many nutritionists to recommend that food supplements are most suitable if they contain a 2:1 ratio of calcium to magnesium, particularly if the diet is low in dairy foods, as only 20–30 per cent of dietary calcium is absorbed.

Five hundred milligrams of calcium and 250 mg of magnesium is a sensible amount with which to supplement the diet, although menopausal woman may choose to take double this dose. People with a normal digestive system wanting to supplement their diet on a long-term basis to maintain bone density should choose Lamberts most popular calcium and magnesium combination product, Osteoguard, or alternatively Dolomite, both available from health food shops. Osteoguard is an ideal product for those concerned with maintaining bone health, as it provides nutrients that research shows work synergistically in bone metabolism, and may also maintain the balance of oestrogen, the natural hormone that helps lay down calcium. Too much calcium can lead to a low level of magnesium. Osteoguard supplies calcium and magnesium at the recommended 2:1 ratio and can be taken alone or in conjunction with high-potency multivitamin formulae.

In osteopathic chiropractic practice can be found a terrific remedy called Joint Mobility Factors, available in health food shops, of which there are two different formulations, one containing glucosamine, which helps to improve the cartilage in the joint, and the other a sulphur-containing compound called MSM. Joint Mobility Factors contains nutrients known to be essential for the proper functioning of the joint system, for example potassium, vitamins B5, B6 and D, magnesium, potassium, alfalfa, bromelain, phenylalanine, devil's claw and yucca. The recommended daily dose of either version of the product is three tablets daily.

Those with osteoporosis often suffer great pain, which may lead to insomnia and depression as well as problems with movement. Other chapters give advice on these areas.

The most popular medical treatment for osteoporosis is synthetic oestrogen, as hormone replacement therapy (HRT), but, as discussed in the chapter on the menopause, this can have many side-effects. Unfortunately, studies indicate that as soon as oestrogen therapy is stopped, bone loss escalates, which means that a woman would have to remain on the oestrogen for a very long time for her bones to be protected by this alone. Phytogen, containing plant-based oestrogen-like substances, is a natural alternative to this; this too is described in the chapter on menopause.

In the forty years during which I have been an osteopath, there have been many times that I have looked for ways of relieving the often severe pain in my patients who really need manipulation, but even soft tissue manipulation carries too great a risk. I will often decide on electro-acupuncture as an initial treatment and then discuss the bone problem. It is for this reason that it is so important to go to a qualified practitioner, be this an osteopath or a chiropractor.

So, there is much that we can do to deal with the problem of osteoporosis and leave us feeling as fabulous as possible. It must not be forgotten that one of the most important things we can do is tell the next generation the facts so that they too can look forward to a fruitful future if they take care of their bodies.

12

How do I cope with insomnia?

Insomnia can become a significant problem as we get older, basically because we need less sleep than we did when we were younger. More than ten million people in the UK suffer from sleep problems, some having done so for many years. Poor sleep patterns lead to an increase in stress-related symptoms and result in a need to relax and escape life's hustle and bustle, as shown by a recent survey which estimated that 270,000 people take time off work as a result of work-related stress. In addition, the Department of Health has estimated that, in 1995, 15.9 million prescriptions were written for sleeping pills and tranquillisers, costing the NHS an enormous, 22.3 million.

Our busy life today suffers from a lack of balance which accounts for an unequal distribution of physical and mental work. We often overtax our minds and do not provide sufficient exercise for our bodies, which consequently diminishes our ability to relax. We cannot rid ourselves of the many problems that haunt us and still subject our already heavily burdened mind to even more stress. Is it any wonder that we cannot fall asleep?

As the quality of our sleep so obviously affects our physical and mental well-being, and as insomnia is one of the most common health problems, this is an area we need to tackle to make the second half of our lives as fulfilling as possible.

First of all, we need to identify whether or not our sleep is of good quality. What are the tests of good and adequate sleep? We may summarise these as follows:

- we should be able to fall asleep reasonably soon after lying down in bed
- we should remain asleep throughout the night, or if we do chance to wake, we should fall asleep again practically immediately
- we should wake in the morning feeling that we have enjoyed our sleep, and be fresh, alert and ready for the new day before us

If we cannot answer positively to these three conditions, sleep is not refreshing us as it naturally should.

And how much sleep should we have? Sleeping, like eating, is a very personal affair. Eight hours may be considered a rough average, but many people keep perfectly well and function efficiently with as little as six, while others need a good nine hours. Our bedtime and time of rising are generally fixed by our need to work, but the aim should be to get to bed at a time that will allow the eight or so hours of sleep necessary for good health.

There are many symptoms of sleeping problems, for example difficulty in getting to sleep, recurrently waking in the night and a generally disturbed sleep. Looking at some of the factors that may contribute to this can help us to prevent or even cure some of these problems. It is agreed by the ablest authorities that sleep is very much a matter of habit, of providing our brain with signals that it is bedtime. The well-known authors Maria and Marcus Webb have written extensively on the subject of sleep and have been of great help to myself and Gloria in writing this book. For example, they have said that it is no secret to parents that children tend to respond positively to bedtime routines. We tend to sleep best in those conditions which the mind has learned to associate with sleep. So it is not uncommon to find that people who sleep amid noise – say, near to a railway shunting station – experience difficulty in sleeping if they are suddenly transplanted to a bedroom where utter quiet reigns. Some may demand complete darkness as a condition of easy sleep, while others prefer a dim light burning all night. Some find difficulty in sleeping if they go to bed unusually early; others find similar difficulty if they retire unusually late – a regular bedtime is important for healthy sleep to keep us feeling fabulous. Sleep is, in short, very much a matter of routine, but while this is natural, bear in mind that it is possible to become too much a slave to mere environment. A relaxed, common-sense, approach is much better, and much more effective, than any frantic attempt to fit into a schedule. Sleep should not be made a matter of anxious concern or of finicky planning.

To make sure you get a good night's sleep, a few simple checks can be made. First, check your mattress, as a poorly supporting mattress can cause discomfort in the night, especially if you suffer from back pain or muscular aches and pains. Remember to turn your mattress once a week to avoid wear in one place; experts have recommended changing it altogether every seven years. Make sure too that your pillow keeps your head in line with your spine.

Next, check the room temperature. Experts recommend a temperature of between 15 and 18°C (60 and 65°F) as being the best temperature for sleeping. If the room is colder than 12 or 13°C (55°F), this may increase the number of highly emotional and unpleasant dreams.

Try to remove anything related to work from your bedroom so that you will be less likely to be reminded of work, and will be able to concentrate on getting a good night's sleep. Some form of exercise or a brisk walk in the late afternoon or early evening can also prove to be beneficial (see also the chapter on exercise). Try, too, not to nap throughout the day.

A warm bath just before going to bed is a wonderful relaxant: anything that recirculates the blood and drives it to the external areas helps to induce sleep, since insomnia is often caused by blood congestion in the brain. Try adding a few drops of relaxing essential oil such as chamomile or lavender to your bath. After the bath, massage your neck and shoulders gently or, even better, get someone else to give you a massage using a relaxing aromatherapy blend. In cases where the nerves have been overtaxed, it is helpful to massage the aching area of the head with the fingertips. This gentle massage generally relaxes tension and results in sleep. A few drops of lavender essential oil on your pillow will also help to give a good night's sleep, or try applying a chamomile compress to the head at bedtime to encourage sleep. Other ways of relaxing – for example, deep breathing – are described later in the chapter as well as in the chapter on exercise.

Sauna baths, once popular in only northern countries, are now accepted in many other areas of the world. In Switzerland and northern Europe, it is common for people in the winter to take a sauna bath and then roll in freshly fallen snow. The claim is that the body's power of resistance becomes greatly strengthened by this exercise. Walking barefoot in the snow and water stamping are other favourite activities. All of these activities cause the blood to be drawn from the brain; when practised before going to bed, this makes restful and wholesome sleep possible. Information on various applications coming in from different countries may benefit us too, since these add variety to the list of already available remedies.

I was greatly surprised to encounter a sauna bath among people living in a Finnish colony in Brazil. What purpose is there for a sauna bath in an area where the temperature reaches 40°C (105°F)? The answer is whatever one is used to seems to become a necessity, which is true for these Finnish people who built their sauna in a hot foreign land, helping them to overcome nostalgia for their homeland. Nevertheless, evenings are cool in the tropics, and thus the sauna bath was a welcome addition to a life pattern developed here. After the sauna bath, a nearby jungle creek tempted us to a cool bathe which stimulated the circulation and helped to provide restful sleep.

A radical approach to inducing sleep is provided in a letter that I recently received from Australia from a former patient. She wrote with great gusto about a book written by Sebastian Kneip, the founder of hydrotherapy, on cold water therapy. Her enthusiasm led her to provide a cold water treatment for her entire family. Her husband, who had been suffering from insomnia for months, had been relieved by applying cold water packs to the back of his head and neck just before going to sleep. One of their daughters, also suffering from insomnia, tried her father's method and was able to fall asleep without any trouble. This provided a spiritual and emotional relief that was of great benefit to her. Various water-based treatments are described in the chapter on exercise.

Many find it possible to put the cares of the day out of mind when going to bed by reading a book, a magazine or some interesting article, which will, if one reads long enough, eventually lead to drowsiness and uninterrupted sleep. Reading in bed is definitely the safest kind of sleep-inducing drug. Today, health books have a wide circulation in every country. The thought that my health books, which are available all over the world, translated into several different languages, could be effective as a sleeping remedy long after I am gone is rather a pleasant one!

If you are suffering from insomnia, it is important also to look at your eating pattern. When I first came to the UK, I told my mother in Holland that Britain was the most wonderful country because you had four meals a day, the fourth meal, supper at nine o'clock being the best; in Holland, we have only three meals, and by six o'clock we have finished the last big meal of the day. This supper, which may consist of crackers and cheese while watching television, is unfortunately often responsible for preventing many people sleeping. Going to bed on a full stomach, especially of cheese and biscuits, which may cause wild dreams, is not the most advisable course of action. The last meal of the day should precede bedtime by three or four hours as it is wrong to expect the stomach to work hard while we sleep. Remember, too, that not only the size of the meal, but also what it consists of is important. A small meal of something that is difficult to digest, such as cheese or other high-protein foods, especially meat, is just as bad as, and perhaps worse than, a large meal. Carbohydrates are preferable to proteins.

Furthermore, lack of sleep may not be entirely due to the late meal: plenty of people omit supper altogether and still fail to sleep. Some people, knowing that they will have little or no supper, eat a large amount of bread at teatime. Like most sedentary people, their digestion is slow, and the indigestible meal at five o'clock keeps them awake just as much as pickles, cucumber, or something equally indigestible eaten at eight o'clock or later. It must be remembered, however, that it is not a good idea to go to bed hungry; in this case, try a light supper of, for example, milk and a couple of biscuits, eaten an hour and a half before bedtime.

You may also have been drinking strong coffee for years. If this is the case, gradually wean yourself off by using a cereal or fruit coffee such as Bambu coffee. This may be difficult at first but your palate will adjust itself to the new taste in a surprisingly short time. In the end, you will be having a harmless drink that will permit you to rest through the night undisturbed. Avoid too, fizzy drinks and teas that contain caffeine. Herbal teas are another enjoyable drink; peppermint can help to stimulate the digestive system, and chamomile will relax your mind.

Soothing herbs include lime flowers, skullcap and borage, while Valerian and Vervain are known for their relaxing properties. Valerian can be obtained in combination with hops as produced by Bioforce. Valerian's effects as a sedative are, however, narcotic, but a drop added to either of the two remedies mentioned will have a calming effect. One good sleeping draught is lemon balm, the effect of which may be increased by the addition of hops. The homeopathic remedy is Avena Sativa (extract of oats). These, taken together, have an excellent sleep-inducing effect, and ready-made preparations are available on the market.

Homeopathic remedies for sleeping problems include coffea, kali phos, and lycopodium for anxiety-related insomnia that leaves you tired in the mornings (see below for more on this). Mountain guides in Switzerland know another good remedy: marmot oil, which can be obtained from many herbalists. A teaspoonful of this taken daily will induce sleep, but as it is not too palatable, it is best taken as gelatine capsules.

In addition to cutting out heavy meals and caffeine-rich drinks, try to avoid smoking as nicotine craving can wake you in the night.

After your evening meal, instead of sitting down to watch television, take a short walk and do some deep breathing exercises, which will be described later on. This will help your digestion, benefit your health and go a long way towards ensuring a good night's sleep. The common sense approach is, as we had said before, best.

Another major culprit affecting the quality of sleep is pain. It may be sensory pain when the body moves during sleep, or pain arising from pressure, which also involves the sympathetic nervous system. The effects of pain during our waking hours are hard enough to bear, but if it disturbs our sleep, it is even more devastating. The body's resources become depleted if the pain continues, so medical advice must be sought. Chronic insomnia and pain may benefit from acupuncture.

But what if you have tried all these suggestions, are counting sheep every night but are still having sleep problems? Some people sleep badly because they think too much about it. Sleep is after all a natural function, as natural as breathing or eating. The moment we begin to make it a matter of desperate and anxious effort, we exacerbate the problem: whenever we become anxious and worried about any body function, we tend to disturb it. A child merely curls up in bed and instinctively sleeps. He does not need to be taught how to sleep; he does not imagine it is a difficult thing. In this way, we may learn wisdom from children.

Other people sleep badly because they rather like it! This may sound simply ridiculous, but it is nonetheless true. We will make this clearer in the chapter that covers getting the best out of life, but we should note here that there are certain people who make insomnia a matter of self-importance.

Another reason is that people sleep poorly because they expect to. They go upstairs with the thought vaguely and dimly at the back of their minds that they will spend another weary sleepless night. Now, the mind has an uncanny way of producing the kind of things it expects so for good functioning, we need a certain measure of quiet confidence that the correct thing will happen. If you have been sleepless one night, take it for granted that when you go to bed you will sleep soundly the next. Trust your own body more confidently; after all, it is only sense that a person who is sleep deprived should go to sleep readily when the chance comes.

A frequent cause of poor sleep is, however, that many people choose night-time to reflect upon every worry, problem and trouble. This is a bad idea: first of all, our reasoning powers are at their lowest ebb in the small hours, so at that time we are least able to think clearly or decide wisely; and in the second place, a good night's rest would do far more for us than fretting and worrying about problems.

It is certainly frustrating not being able to go to sleep in spite of being tired, and it is probably even worse to lie awake for hours because the tensions of the day are transformed at night into problems of insurmountable magnitude. Unpleasant daytime experiences prevent sleep and create a state of depression, and the wheels of the mind, which are supposed to stand still during the night, turn faster and faster. Suffering from restlessness, the individual tosses, and finally, in order to put an end to the suffering, reaches for a sleeping pill to overcome the insomnia. This, of course, is the most inappropriate choice, for in no time, if this habit continues, he or she will have developed a dependence on this crutch. This destroys the body's ability to react and respond in a natural way, and the continued use of sleep-inducing drugs, whether or not they are habit-forming, has a destructive effect that can be far reaching. It is far more important and wiser to isolate the cause of the problem that keeps us awake; by resolving it, we will eventually restore our ability to sleep.

And what of those people who are not aware of sleeping badly but who wake feeling anything but refreshed and certainly not ready for the day? They wake up tired, yet they may have spent ten hours in bed and have actually slept for most of that time. Such people are loathe to get up. And when they do come down to breakfast, they are irritable, moody and snappish. Why is this? This will be explored more fully in the chapter on how to get the best out of life; suffice it to say for the moment that in all such cases there is something deep seated in the mind that, even during sleep, worries and irritates. This may be a problem or task that has been avoided, or more rarely, a sense of guilt, which, while not actually preventing sleep, robs us of its beneficial and recuperative effects. As Abraham Lincoln once said, 'You have to sleep with your conscience'; a troubled conscience is a bad bed-fellow.

There are three ways in which one can generally dispel worries at night. The first is to decide to tackle the problem that is worrying you at a definite time the next day and to forget it in the meantime; it is surprising how effective a self-promise to act at a later date can be. The second strategy is not just to put the worry out of the mind, but to replace it with something more attractive – your next holiday, for example. The third method is preparing ourselves by relaxing before we go to bed.

Sleep is a sort of prolonged relaxation, but such relaxation cannot be sustained for a lengthy period, whereas sleep can be enjoyed for hours at a stretch. The close relationship between the two is, however, proved by the fact that most people who have become to some degree proficient in systematic relaxation find it quite usual to fall asleep when relaxation is prolonged beyond a fairly short period of ten minutes or so. There is no better way of establishing the habit of sound, healthy sleep, night by night, than a few moments spent daily in systematic relaxation – any form of relaxation that enables you to sleep.

A few simple exercises may help while you are lying in bed. First, put your left hand just below your navel and place your right hand on top of this. Breathe deeply through your mouth into your abdomen, and then slowly exhale through your nose. Repeat this until you feel completely relaxed and sleepy. An alternative is the Arti Arti exercise: move your arms and feet up and down rhythmically and close your eyes. Soon you will feel very relaxed. My book *Body Energy* outlines a few more exercises.

One of the most powerful methods of achieving relaxation lies in the control of our breathing, and we are fortunate that nature has provided us with our own in-built stress-buster. Even the most stressed can take advantage of this when they know how. Incredibly, your breathing rate will be changed in just seconds, although, of course, it initially takes time and effort to perfect the technique. The great shame is that, for most of us, this in-built method of stress control remains on the whole untapped. The majority have lost the ability to breathe naturally, that is, deeply and slowly. The faster and shallower our breathing becomes, the more harassed and fraught we feel.

Next time you have the opportunity, watch how a healthy child breathes, especially when asleep (remembering that a baby breathes at a much faster pace). The breaths are regular, slow and deep, coming from somewhere between the lower chest and the abdomen. If the child is dreaming, his or her breathing occasionally quickens and comes from the upper chest, although it quickly returns to the steady, slow rhythmical pattern. This is what you should be aiming to achieve. When stressed, your breathing will quicken and come from your upper chest. This will dramatically alter the level of the gases in your blood, and you will be forced to breathe even more quickly to gain the oxygen you need. This leads to symptoms of light-headedness and dizziness, the only way to stop this vicious cycle in its tracks being to force yourself to slow your breathing down. When relearning to breathe properly or even normally, the simplest method is to overexaggerate the normal breathing pattern. This will make it easier to highlight where the breath is coming from so that it can easily be changed and fine-tuned.

First, lie in a quiet room where you are unlikely to be distracted. Place one hand on your abdomen and your other on your upper chest. Take a slow deep breath in through your nose, making sure it bypasses the upper hand so that it reaches the lower hand, on your upper abdomen. Hold the breath for a few seconds and then slowly control the breath as you exhale through your mouth. Wait for a couple of seconds before repeating the process. Initially, practise this for only five breaths as, depending on how poor your breathing has become, it may leave you feeling light-headed. Some people will have misused their breathing so badly that their diaphragm will only slowly begin to judder back into action.

If you are to use this system of stress relief properly, it is worth practising daily so that you learn totally to control your breathing. This does not mean spending hours each day getting it right. In fact, it is detrimental to do this, as you may hyperventilate (contributing to an alteration in the balance of oxygen and carbon dioxide in the blood); pressure from your daily schedule will also hamper you. Just a few minutes of deep breathing on rising will enable you to start the day calm and full of energy, and at the close of the day ensure that you enjoy a full and restful night's sleep.

It will obviously take time to re-establish a normal breathing pattern, but just remember that it will be worth it in the end, when you are faced with a tense situation and need a cool head. Once you have perfected this technique, you can move onto other, more specific techniques; my book *Stress and Nervous Disorders* may give you a few ideas.

Using the same basic breathing method outlined earlier, count one mentally in your head on every breath out. The aim is to reach five; although this sounds simple, very few people manage to achieve a score of above three. This is because every time you have an incoming thought, you have to return to one again.

Apart from offering an alternative to counting sheep, this technique has a number of benefits. It will allow you to focus your mind, emptying it of all thoughts, but more importantly will allow you to discover what may really be troubling you. Initially, trivial thoughts will creep in, such as what you are going to prepare for dinner or whether you have remembered to set your alarm clock. The thoughts that occur often are similar to those which wake you in the middle of the night. Keep a pen and paper beside you (now, as well as at night), and write down each incoming thought. This way you can then forget about it and it will not keep nagging you and disturbing you. After doing this over a period of time, the more serious worries start to emerge. Again, write them down. Don't try to make sense of them at this moment, but carry on with your relaxation and deal with them at a more convenient time.

If you require clarity of mind, a breathing technique that has been used since ancient times is to exhale through both nostrils individually. This technique can also be effective for sinus problems. Place a finger over your right nostril and slowly breathe in. Then, also put a finger over your left nostril, holding the breath for a couple of seconds, before releasing your finger from your right nostril and breathing out. Repeat this a few times.

If tension seems to be related to a forthcoming event such as an exam, using your breathing with specific visual imagination might not only relieve your anxiety, but also ensure that you perform to the best of your ability. Lie in a quiet room and imagine yourself preparing for the forthcoming event. Visualise yourself on the day – getting to the exam room a few minutes before the exam, turning the paper over, reading it and then finally doing the exam. Imagine your feelings afterwards. If at any time your breathing increases, focus on that point; perhaps it is when you turn the paper over. What is it that is worrying you? Try to slow your breathing down. Then, keep replaying that part until your breathing stays at a relaxed rate. Many people have found this technique invaluable when they are prone to panic: common situations include flying, job interviews and confrontations with colleagues or friends.

So remember the following when trying to ensure regular sound sleep:

- Sleep is not difficult: it is the most natural thing in the world.
- If you suffer from poor sleep, don't talk about it – dwelling on the problem will only reinforce it in your mind.
- Acquire the art of switching your mind to pleasant thoughts. Leave your worries and problems resolutely outside the bedroom door.
- Trust your own body. Your body will behave better if you treat it with a little confidence.

- Do not rely on drugs. If you have been in the habit of using them, cut down gradually. Relaxation and auto-suggestion can do more for you than medication.
- Go to sleep with the thought that you will get up in the morning feeling well, fresh and keenly alive. Let your last thoughts be of peace and calm, generous goodwill to all the world, quietness, confidence and serenity.

13

How do I care for my partner?

Fact – women live longer than men. Fact – men live longer if they are in a married or secure relationship. As a woman, I think it's fair to say that most of us are born nurturers, so caring for the people around us should come naturally and instinctively. We have all heard the expression 'what you sow is what you reap', so if we want to create a sense of well-being in our lives, it follows we have to lay the foundation and sow the seeds of caring and happiness. I know, of course, that some women will say, in these days of equality, 'What about me? I need a lot of nurturing too.' We *all* do, but, in the main, women naturally appear to be the constant and consistent carers, whether of a child, a husband or a parent.

In this chapter, we are looking at caring for our partner in life. I now regard myself as being very fortunate in that, having gone through a divorce from a man I was married to for over twenty years, I ended up meeting Stephen Way, now my husband, when I was aged around fifty-three and he a year older. We were great friends for about a year before our relationship grew, for which I am very grateful, because we knew how much we genuinely liked and respected each other before the sexual side of our relationship developed.

We got married five years later and had had only about ten months of wedded bliss before Stephen suffered a minor heart attack totally out of the blue. This occurred in a man who was fit and strong, in many ways the last person on earth I would have expected it to happen to.

Apart from the obvious worry and anxiety this situation produces, it throws a relationship onto a different and extra level. 'Caring and nurturing' really comes into its own where life is being threatened. And what a learning curve it has been for me as well. To have someone and something so treasured and then nearly to have him taken away certainly sharpens the senses and makes one appreciate literally every second.

Fortunately, Stephen is one of the lucky ones in many ways, has had a timely warning and will be regularly monitored, but in the process we have both learned so much about caring for each other not only a day-to-day basis, but also on a practical level, and about some of the do's and don'ts of diet, of exercise and vitamin supplements. I now believe that when one person in the relationship is put under severe pressure, it helps if the other joins in with the regime of the right food, the routine of exercise and any adjustments of lifestyle necessary, and I truly believe that, in supporting Stephen in his new regime, I have benefited in so many ways and been re-educated.

Every relationship is one of give and take, and compromise. I like what Deepak Chopra, the philosopher, says, that 'giving to each other engenders receiving, and receiving engenders giving. What you give out some how comes back.' Chopra goes on to say that receiving is the same thing as giving because both are different aspects of the flow of love and energy, and if you stop the flow of either, you interfere with nature's balance and intelligence.

Anything which is of value in your life only multiplies when it is given with love. If you give grudgingly, there is no energy behind that giving. Your intention should always be to create happiness for both the giver and receiver, because happiness is life supporting and life sustaining. This energy between two people is what we all have to aspire to within any relationship.

As this book is about how we feel after fifty, it is probably worth putting the spotlight generally on relationships, as we move into that 'third period' of our lives. Many worry about the atmosphere within a household when the children grow up and move out into their own worlds. I feel that it is almost like those teenage years all over again, a certain kind of freedom to do all the things you have not had time for within a busy family household. Not having to be there to pick children up from school or to make their dinner spot on time gives you both the freedom to be able to act spontaneously without the restrictions of being hands-on parents. There is now precious time together – to take up that game of golf you have been promising yourself, to go on holiday at the last minute, to learn a new language, or just to mooch about enjoying the new-found freedom.

In conclusion, we are all travellers on our journey of life; we have stopped for a period of time to encounter each other, to meet, to love, to share. These are precious moments of time, but they are transient. However, if we share with caring, lightheartedness, and love, we will create abundance and joy for each other, and this moment will then have been worthwhile.

Caring is a very important aspect of a relationship. When Gloria chose this chapter, the first consideration that came to my mind was the element of care within a partnership. We should stop and consider how much we show that we care for our partner. How unselfish are we? And how much effort do we go to in putting our partners before ourselves?

After a television programme that Gloria and I had recorded together, I received a very interesting letter. The writer said that, most of the time, she felt simply awful and not at all the person she really believed herself to be, not at all fabulous. She had a great longing to regain her normal life, yet upon wakening in the morning was saying to herself, 'Oh no, not another day.' Her appetite had suffered, she was experiencing nervous anxiety, but she believed that she had no reason at all to be feeling these symptoms. The writer said that she loved her job, yet felt so nervous about going to work that she would often cry. At times she felt completely exhausted and was engulfed in anxiety. She had consulted her GP, counsellors and numerous other practitioners, who only seemed to give her antidepressant after antidepressant.

Finally, the reader felt that the breakdown in her personality was alienating her husband. She had lost all interest in a sexual relationship with her husband and felt that they were very quickly drifting apart. As a result she was terrified that they would end up leading separate lives.

I read through this letter when the title of this chapter came to mind; partnership is valuable in many ways. I also remember a couple who for ten years faithfully listened to the Radio 2 show that Gloria and I did together. Over this time, I built up a very good relationship with many of my patients, and whenever a diamond wedding anniversary arises, I endeavour to attend these very special occasions. This particular couple, whom I have known for almost thirty-two years, are the happiest couple that I have ever come across. Their relationship is as strong as it was when they first met. They care for each other and love each other; as he once said, 'I see my marriage as a limited company with equal rights and equal cares to make it work and prosper'. Both are quite youthful for their age, and it is obvious that a harmonious relationship pays out enormous dividends and bonuses right to the very end. In the beginning, it may well be all sunshine and romantic moonlight, but, once the marriage has gone on for a few years, little niggles and worries, together with daily familiarity, can give rise to some problems.

It is at this time that one should heed these little warning signs. I recently read that most divorces occur around the three-year or eleven-year period, or some time after twenty-five years. Whether or not these statistics are valid, one thing is certain: you certainly learn to know each other inside out after a few years. Little irritations can begin to replace endearing habits, and these can build up to such a point that a separation or divorce can ensue.

Personally, I must have the most understanding wife in the world, and when I was thinking about this chapter, it crossed my mind that I actually have no right whatsoever to advocate the best ways of caring for a partner as I am very seldom at home and often away on business. Unfortunately, other people are not as understanding as my wife, and friction then arises within the relationship.

Give and take is very important. It is purely a matter of discussion and communication, which is probably one of the most important elements of a successful relationship. We should stop and consider how often we really do talk to and discuss important issues with our partners.

The other day a lady came to the clinic. She appeared very unkempt in appearance and quite upset, almost suffocating in her own worries. Her husband had taken off with his secretary and she felt that he no longer found her attractive as she was over fifty. As a result of the menopause, their sex life had deteriorated, and her husband had apparently sought opportunities elsewhere. She confided that she would do anything at all to regain her husband and save her marriage.

I first told her that she should take a good look at herself and decide whether she liked what she saw. If not, there were several things that she could do to help herself. Her appearance gave the impressions that she did not care for herself. If she thought back to when she first met her husband, she remembered that she paid attention to her personal appearance and cared about herself. By regaining pride in herself and in her appearance, her husband could be reminded of the attractive girl he first met.

I gave this lady a few remedies to help build up her confidence, one of which – Female Essence – would help to eliminate her jealousy and insecurity. I also gave her ginseng to help re-energise her and a course of Woman Power to resurrect her desire for a physical relationship. These remedies help to restore the hormonal balance and provide sufficient vitamins and minerals to support the nervous system.

The lady returned two weeks later and reported that the situation had improved; indeed, she was very hopeful that things would work out between her and her husband. Fortunately, they did: upon sitting down and communicating their individual worries and concerns, they agreed to reunite.

Different experiences within a relationship will have differing effects on each partner. These experiences will not only affect the physical body, but also the emotional body. To sit down and discuss your grievances is not enough: each partner has a responsibility to understand how events are affecting the other and to decide how best to solve the problems with which they are faced. It is highly surprising how much easier it is to understand a partner's actions if you are determined to be positive. Taking a negative and pessimistic approach, believing that all is lost, is a defeatist attitude.

Honesty is a very important element in a relationship. Dishonesty will always lead to a breakdown of trust and respect, and will ultimately lead to the destruction of what may have been a good relationship. To lie about misdemeanours will not lead to a positive resolution of the problem. Being honest enables both partners to learn from the experience.

Body and soul can often come into conflict. Harmony between the physical and the emotional body will bring forth the positive energy for interaction between the two. As we have suggested in another chapter, the harmonious energy within our relationships is of utmost importance. We have all experienced those wonderful moments when the bio-energies between two people are so perfect that you feel you are in heaven. This is something that a couple can work on. Such energies are not there all the time, and life is certainly not always paradise, but it is wonderful when we can work at our relationships and discover the key to resolving the problems that occur. Communication often allows situations to resolve themselves.

Energy is powerful; it exists within every one of us, vibrating out towards others. Like ripples, the positive thoughts and actions emanate outwards, affecting your surroundings. When you balance the cosmic energies that have been given to you, these will vibrate between you and your partner. Therefore, the reflection of these vibrations will affect both of you, and you have a responsibility to maintain this equilibrium. We have only just begun to scrape the surface of the potential power of the energy within us all. Daily, in my work, I realise that our personal energy and how we maintain its balance is very much up to the individual. No-one else can do it for you: the responsibility is yours alone.

Positive action always overcomes negative action. Our unconscious mind will develop if we allow the energy within us to flow and vibrate outwards. The subconscious mind, which we do not really know much about, except that it generates positive cosmic energy that vibrates through us, will help in the most difficult circumstances of life. When problems arise and a partner does not understand, the subconscious mind will help to restore the disturbed energy within us.

I saw an example of this in a relationship that had come to

a complete end. Both partners had tried very hard to maintain harmony, but eventually they gave up trying and admitted defeat. Although they fought very hard against each other, they were both still longing to find the inner peace that would restore the harmony and balance of their relationship. Deep down, they still cared for each other and did not wish the relationship to end. They both had one consideration uppermost in their minds – their children. They desperately wanted to bring their children up in a secure and loving environment, and they realised that in order to do so, they would have to restore the balance and harmony that had once existed between them. They agreed to unconditionally share and care for each other, and they ultimately managed to regain a great deal of what they thought had deserted them.

Another couple who were experiencing great strain and tension as a result of illness received help from several remedies. For example, Avena Sativa, along with Neuroforce, can help to provide a positive attitude. Concentration Essence also helps to balance our energies, promoting harmony and mental clarity. All of these remedies can be bought in health food shops.

In caring for our partner, we must remember to live in harmony. Each and every event in our lives, when they are combined, give us a message or a purpose. Love is vital in every relationship and if there is caring, there is love. Show that you love each other by unexpected invitations to dinner, a surprise bunch of flowers, even writing a letter describing your appreciation and feelings. These small gestures are very important in maintaining a mutually supportive and loving relationship.

It may be that the over-fifties do not have the same problems as under-fifties. The over-fifties have learned from past experiences how to live harmoniously together or, in some cases, that it is better for both to go their separate ways. It is no good if a marriage or partnership becomes a millstone around the neck. This amounts to killing each other slowly and is a very destructive process. When I look back at marriages that I have seen held together for the children's sake, I see that they have been no more than a living hell for the partners and, at times, for the children too.

It is no good continuing with a destructive relationship. It may sometimes be helpful separating from each other and evaluating your wants, desires and expectations. Sometimes you will realise that you do not want to lose your partner and that you still care for them. Sometimes such separations can point towards an alternative route that will benefit both parties. Caring is sharing, as the saying goes. By sharing, most things we do are of the greatest benefit. Caring for each other and talking about everyday experiences is important.

Emotions and feelings that are shared always result in some sort of positive action. One lady told me the other day that her marriage had started wonderfully, but then her husband started to hide certain things. He didn't want to discuss business matters with her and then went on to hide financial mistakes that he had made; at long last, he was virtually leading a secret life. Sadly, this led to the end of the relationship. People often claim to have wasted too much time on a relationship and are often filled with regret. It is no good sitting down and regretting what might have been; what matters is a positive decision is made that will benefit both the present and the future.

I heard a very similar story from a lady who had lived with her partner for nearly thirty years. He promised her that he would marry her when he had time. When he had obtained all that he wanted from her, including her savings and bank account numbers, he left, sneaking away and leaving her a letter telling her that their relationship was over. This woman sat and sobbed in front of me. I told her that she was very lucky that she had not married him, as the relationship was a one-sided affair with no hope of a future.

Sometimes in a relationship, one partner is totally powerless and doesn't know how to take action. If love is there, the strengthening energies will arise. With balanced vibrations of energies, perfection almost exists. Love will supply understanding. Love will show that a partnership is equal. A relationship that has grown through caring is instinctively understood by two people in a truly motivational and creative exercise.

All committed partnerships will work. I once read that marriage is a partnership not a dictatorship; when I came from Holland to Great Britain I saw many dictatorships. In some areas of the country, men are honoured as a king on a throne and the wife is often less than a slave. I saw the most unhappy relationships with the men being dominant. One has to realise that a partnership is an equal relationship and should work accordingly.

Every day we are given a great abundance of energy that we can work with. To see the positive energy is sometimes difficult, especially if one tends towards a negative outlook. Barriers are often erected, and we are unable to observe our relationship clearly or see the role that both partners are playing. We forget to talk and we do not see the possibilities.

Energy in our body not only vibrates, but also give life through harmony of the cells directing the negatives towards the positives. Negative never looks for positive, yet positive always looks for negative. By discovering this, you will probably find a new exciting feeling of caring within a relationship that will generate happiness. If we think positively that we will care for our partner, we will, and with this caring we will not only feel fabulous but will be repaid with happiness that we may have previously have missed out on.

Energy between two partners is most important. To be on the same wavelength is vital for a successful partnership. This mutual energy that can sometimes by seen in an ideal partnership and is often of terrific encouragement to those who have found themselves in unhappy or destructive relationships. Caring for each other within a loving relationship will enable you to get through the ups and downs, but also will encourage friendship to grow. Without friendship, there is without doubt a break that sometimes cannot be healed.

When we lost that real feeling that we once had for our partner, we stop caring. Then comes the thought 'Where do I go from here?' It is always important to sit down, think about the various possibilities and write down 'Where have I gone wrong? Has my business taken over, has my family taken over, is my social life taking over?' If we want a finely balanced relationship, it is important to look at all the factors that contribute to it – otherwise you will not only lose the security, but also the trust that you had in your partner. It is quite amazing that there are a whole host of individual senses pointing us in the right direction towards that path. Finding the balance is therefore important.

Caring for a partner means unconditionally giving and receiving an energy that flows between partners ensuring happiness and contentment. Should you awake feeling sad and deflated, you should do your best to resolve the situation as best you can. No sympathy is deserved by those who do not attempt to understand their partner. There are a few things that should be done, and you should prioritise in each situation.

When I wrote the book *Inner Harmony*, I received many letters from people saying that they had the lost harmony within their relationship, sometimes as a result of shocking and unforgivable acts of betrayal. These people were fearful, and I often wonder how it is possible for two people who once loved each other to end up being so hurtful. There is always an element of pain, and if I see that a situation is going nowhere, I encourage change. I emphasise that it is necessary to observe and assess the realistic expectations and possibilities of a relationship. Changes may be necessary so you can care for your partner.

The other day, I saw a couple who had been happily married for a number of years. They had shared a lot of sorrow, which resulted in bringing them closer. However, something happened in their life that basically caused them not to care for each other any more. There were health problems involved and I was able to help both of them. They then asked if I could help them with their relationship problems. They had missed some very good opportunities for sorting out their difficulties. Sometimes our potential and our opportunities are unknown to us, but yet they lie just around the corner waiting to be discovered. Asking each other or someone you trust, or even prayer and meditation, can help to reveal that hidden potential at an unexpected time.

There is another major factor that we have to address in a relationship. Breaking a habit is not easy, and often caring for your partner means breaking certain habits. In any partnership, one partner's bad habits will annoy the other, these sometimes being very difficult to eliminate. It takes a great deal of concentration and mental effort. Habits are not controlled so much as they tend to control you. If you let yourself drift without any mental effort in the direction you are taking, you will form habits along the path of least resistance, and unless you subject yourself to severe discipline, you will drift from bad to worse. It is easier to form a good habit than to break a bad one, and habits can only be controlled by a lot of mental effort. You must act efficiently and discipline yourself to create a habit that is more satisfactory than the one which annoys your partner. Concentrate on this new habit and make sure it replaces the bad one. Doing just this is one way of showing you care.

When I came to Britain in 1970, it seemed that, in such a permissive society, a lot of things were allowed but adultery was not. Over forty thousand couples a year quote adultery as grounds for divorce. This reflects a considerable level of discontent, and is not very different from the situation in Holland. Yet there are sometimes reasons for adultery occurring. Of the many couples with whom I have been in touch over the years, whom I have helped to steer away from the option of divorce, the main reason was carelessness.

I remember helping a couple of which the wife had had an affair that only came to light a number of years later. Unfortunately, there was little that I could do at this point. The couple eventually came to the conclusion that they wished to give their relationship another chance. I met them twenty years later and found them to be the happiest of couples. The affair had resulted in them both striving to understand and communicate with each other more effectively, becoming more tolerant of each other.

Counsellors say that there is really no way of determining whether this happens more often with women or men; it is said that 60 per cent of men and 40 per cent of women will have an affair. Hurt, anger and a deep sense of betrayal are often the inevitable emotions when discovering that the person you love is secretly conducting an affair. I have also noticed that such a situation can initiate a new beginning in a relationship as problems brought into the open are faced and resolved, leading to a reunion and resulting in a better relationship. Basically, it is the affection communicated between two people, rather than the sexual relationship, that is more important. There are times when a marriage can be difficult and strained, probably more often before the age of fifty, although we should be aware of it at any age. Everybody's experience is different, and to fall passionately in love does not always guarantee a happy marriage. Communication, talking, recognising problems as they arise and being able to discuss them is an excellent basis for maintaining a caring, affectionate partnership.

The 'retirement' years can be ones in which we can really enjoy sharing life with our partner, without the ongoing demands of employment and duty. Caring, sharing and communicating will allow us to make the most of this special time together.

14

How do I keep my love life going?

It is often said that women are the weaker sex, a statement that has intrigued me over the years. Where does the saying come from, and why should a woman be considered to be weaker than a man? Are any differences apparent that might affect how we age and relate to each other? Can our relationship continue to be as physical as it once was?

Back in 1928 in Amsterdam, women were allowed to participate in the 800 metres run for the first time. Before this, it had been decided that women would not be able to withstand the course and complete the run as it would be too arduous for them. Women were only allowed to participate in the Olympic Marathon in 1984. Women, like men, are fast walkers, but men are basically harder walkers: the fastest woman in the marathon was fifteen minutes behind her male counterpart. This also comes to the fore in swimming.

In other sports, however, some women are quicker than men, and it appears that women will feature more predominantly in sports than men in the future, as they are tending to catch up with men. If a woman trains in her sport, she often has better stamina and tires less easily than a man.

The obvious difference between men and women – apart from their chromosomal make-up – is that women are smaller in stature. Their bones are smaller, their shoulders narrower and their rib cage shorter. However, their neck tends to be longer and slimmer, the joints being more flexible. Men are usually 10 per cent taller, but women tend to be heavier in comparison.

A woman also has the ability to carry and bear a child, made easier by her more flexible joints. However, this ability is accompanied by symptoms associated with the menstrual cycle, as well as the menopause, as described in another chapter. The hormones involved are, however, what gives her her special attractiveness and charm. (*Ginkgo biloba* extract and Siberian ginseng may be of help here.) A woman may continue to develop sexually even up until the age of forty.

The immune system of men is not as strong as that of women, so men are at a greater risk of developing cancer or contracting infections than women. However, the *auto*immune response – the action of the immune system against the body itself – is stronger than that in a man, so women are more likely to develop autoimmune problems.

A woman's digestive system is much slower than a man's. Alcohol also affects women twice as strongly as men, which is why women tend to suffer more from liver cirrhosis.

The forecast of a general lifespan is seventy-five years for a man and eighty-two years for a woman. In the year 2050, it is estimated that is will be eighty years for a man and eighty-three for a woman. The general and most common causes of death for both are cardiovascular problems and cancer, with breast cancer considerably more common in women then men, cancer of the cervix obviously exclusive to women, and that of the prostate to men.

Overall, a woman's senses are more finely attuned. Colour blindness affects one man in eight, whereas only one woman in two hundred or so suffer from this. A woman is also lucky in that her hearing is better than a man's. Women are also more perceptive and more sensitive.

Women are much more emotional than men, and as a result have more empathy. They tend to be more patient and are basically better at dealing with emotional issues.

Overall, however, women are no longer being labelled 'the weaker sex'. In the American army, for example, it is interesting to see that in the six months during which men and women receive their training after joining, women are just as fit as their male counterparts.

As men and women grow older, however, problems may arise that affect their fitness in different ways, and have a knock-on effect on their sex lives. When a woman goes through the menopause, hormonal and physiological changes in her body can trigger off alterations in both her health (see the chapters on the menopause and osteoporosis) and her libido. Every woman differs in these changes, and will differ in her ability to respond sexually, as well as in her sexual desire. Other factors, for example depression and medical problems, may contribute to the difficulties that she experiences, as may emotional stress and anxiety, which can have a direct bearing on a woman's sexual desire. Marital problems or a failure to address properly menopausal symptoms may also cause a drop in sexual desire. In contrast, other women find that their capacity for sexual desire and enjoyment returns after the menopause, some even experiencing an abrupt increase or sharp decrease in their libido.

The menopause does not cause women to age faster, but we cannot ignore the fact that it brings many complex emotional and physiological changes. Older organs are less resistant to stress than younger organs. Maintaining a positive outlook is a major factor in being able to cope psychologically and physically with these changes. It is of the utmost importance to maintain a positive and optimistic outlook on life. There are many tools and opportunities that can be used to achieve a happy and trouble-free transition through this time of life. It should not be a case of saying to yourself, 'I am getting old'. Instead, you should be asking, 'How can I keep young?' No matter what age we are, we should all endeavour to appear well and attractive to others, energy and vitality being major factors in maintaining an attractive personality.

If problems do arise, remedies such as Woman Power from Michael's can help a woman's flagging libido. There is no reason why a regular sexual relationship cannot continue well into old age if both partners' general health allows.

Men encounter somewhat different problems once they reach their sixties and seventies, leaving women more likely than men to be able to enjoy sex in their later years. Although we are not looking at old age specifically in this book, it is wise to be aware of the problems that we may begin to face later in life. Men commonly develop problems with their prostate gland, the gland that surrounds the neck of the bladder and produces one of the constituents of semen. Because of its position, any growth in size of the gland tends to show up as problems with urination, for example excessive night-time urination, painful or difficult urination, a decreased urine flow or an inability to empty the bladder. This can lead to anxiety and a decreased sexual drive.

Unfortunately, prostate cancer is a disease of which many men should be more aware. In 1993, there were 165,000 cases of prostate cancer reported in the USA with 35,000 deaths. Because of the risk of this, any symptoms should immediately be reported to a doctor. What is more likely to be found than a tumour, however, is a condition known as benign prostatic hypertrophy (BPH), or enlarged prostate, the incidence of which is rising. It is estimated that 50 per cent of men in the USA aged fifty and over suffer from BPH.

As prostatic illness becomes more common, concern and health awareness among men is also increasing. Fortunately, a natural herbal extract, saw palmetto, has been shown to treat the symptoms of BPH safely and effectively. This is, according to Professor Varro Tyler of Purdue University, one of the top ten phytomedicines in Western Europe. In Germany, standardised saw palmetto is an approved phytomedicine for BPH.

The oil from the berries that grow on the saw palmetto plant contains sterols that have been shown to have important oestrogenic activity. Countless medical trials have evaluated the effectiveness of saw palmetto oil extract and found it to be effective in the treatment of BPH. There are no safety concerns associated with the short- or long-term use of standardised saw palmetto berry extract, and saw palmetto does not produce some of the adverse side-effects, namely impotence, associated with drugs conventionally used for BPH, such as the anti-androgen Proscar (finasteride).

In the UK, saw palmetto is available as a liquid preparation of fresh extract, and can be obtained from health food stores.

A worrying problem suffered by many men is that of impotence. The term 'impotence' has traditionally been used to signify the inability of the male to attain or maintain an erection of the penis sufficient to permit satisfactory sexual intercourse. Impotence is in most circumstances more precisely referred to as 'erectile dysfunction' as this term differentiates itself from loss of libido, premature ejaculation or an inability to achieve an orgasm.

An estimated 10-20 million men suffer from erectile dysfunction, a number that is expected to increase dramatically as the median age of the population increases. Currently, erectile dysfunction is thought to affect over 25 per cent of men over the age of fifty. Although the frequency increases with age, it must be stressed that ageing itself is not a cause of impotence. Although the amount and force of the ejaculation as well as the need to ejaculate decreases with age, the capacity for erection is retained: men are capable of retaining their sexual virility well into their eighties.

Erectile dysfunction may be caused by organic (physical) or psychogenic factors, in the overwhelming majority of cases the former. In fact, in men over the age of fifty, physical causes are responsible for erectile dysfunction in over 90 per cent of cases. Atherosclerosis of the penile artery is the primary cause of impotence in nearly half the men over the age of fifty who have erectile dysfunction.

As a result of all the media hype, many men are keen to try the drug Viagra, but this is not the only option available when this problem occurs. Viagra has several bad side-effects – indigestion, headaches, visual disturbances and even a prolonged erection – so I would advise that several other options be considered rather than immediately resorting to it. Apart from anything else, your doctor will prescribe Viagra only when it is medically necessary, for example in multiple sclerosis or severe pelvic injury; otherwise it is not available on the NHS.

On should of course start by looking at general measures to help the problem:

- consume a diet that focuses on whole, unprocessed foods (whole grains, legumes, vegetables, fruits, nuts and seeds)
- eliminate alcohol, caffeine and sugar
- identify and control any food allergies

- take regular exercise
- perform a relaxation exercise (deep breathing, meditation, visualisation, etc.) for ten to fifteen minutes each day
- drink at least 1.4 litres (2.5 pints) of water daily

A good remedy for impotence is the combination of Masculex (see below; available from health food shops) at a dose of two tablets twice a day, along with one capsule of ginkgo phytosome twice a day, which can be very effective. The remedy *Ginkgo biloba* extract, at a dose of fifteen drops twice a day, can also be beneficial.

Masculex has been formulated by the company Enzymatic Therapy as a comprehensive supplement for active men of all ages. It was specifically designed to support male glandular function. Some of the valuable ingredients in this supplement are:

Vitamin E (d-alpha-tocopherol)

The term 'tocopherol' comes from the Greek words meaning 'off-spring' and 'to bear'; hence, tocopherol literally means 'to bear children'. Vitamin E is also a valuable anti-oxidant and supports the immune system.

Muira Puama

This herb, which is little known but boasts its exotic origins in Brazil, was shown in a recent French study to be clinically effective in improving sexual function in some patients. Its Brazilian name is 'potency wood', which suggests that the locals didn't need to hear the verdict of the French team before recognising its value in this arena. Researchers believe that this herb influences the patient both psychologically and physically.

Liquid liver fractions

Liver is the richest natural source of many vitamins and minerals. A key benefit of liver extracts occurs because the liver is the most important organ of metabolism – when liver function improves, metabolism improves. An improved metabolism creates high energy levels and a greater feeling of health and well-being, of feeling fabulous. Liquid liver extracts are a remarkable tonic for well-being.

Saw palmetto

This constituent, which we mentioned above, comes from a small palm tree native to the West Indies and the Atlantic coast of North America. The American Indians administered the berries of this plant to men in order to increase the function of their testicles and to relieve irritation of the mucous membranes, particularly those of the genitourinary tract and prostate. Many herbalists consider it to be an aphrodisiac.

Cola nut extract (containing 4.8mg of caffeine)

This is a natural energising dietary supplement.

Panax ginseng

In studies with animals, sperm formation and testosterone level increased with ginseng administration, and increased sexual activity and mating behaviour were observed. This herb is also a good tonic for general well-being and energy level.

Ginkgo biloba

Ginkgo, a valuable herb for increasing both blood flow and oxygen to many tissues, is described more fully in the chapter of the menopause.

All this assumes, of course, that the couple are willing to admit that there is a problem and willing to do something about it, but I sometimes see patients who are enduring sexual problems through lack of knowledge or lack of communication. These problems can arise from several different areas. Some women think that their clitoris is the wrong size or shape, and men may think that their penis is too small, whether erect or not. These seemingly small problems can result in a great deal of anxiety and hence affect sexual performance. Sometimes women have deep-seated fears concerning the vagina and become fearful of penetration. Some men think that they are incapable of fully satisfying a woman. These misunderstandings and fears, if handled correctly and patiently, can be resolved, and normal happy sexual activity can be fully enjoyed.

Many sexual problems and the resulting difficulties arise from ignorance of the facts of life, as well as ignorance of the physiological make-up of our bodies. To prevent this, everyone should be aware of his or her own physiological and physical make-up. Sex should not be perceived as an area of dark secrets; sexuality is an essential part of our make-up, and sexual activity is part and parcel of our lives.

I sometimes come across older couples who are unaware of many of the facts surrounding sexual physiology and activity. Many of the older generation view sex as an undesirable and 'dodgy' subject that should not be given any thought and consideration, but for them the attainment of a fully satisfying sex life is perfectly possible. Enjoying a close and physical relationship with the person you love is one of the most enjoyable and intimate ways of expressing your emotions, and it is a part of a relationship that should be respected and cherished. The subject of sex should not be a 'no-go' area or a closed book for discussion between two partners. Instead, it should be discussed openly.

Sadly, many men and women are unable to find the correct means of communicating their sexual needs, desires and problems within their relationships. Knowledge that is combined with love, respect and maturity will help to support and encourage a lasting and satisfactory sexual relationship.

Many couples experience sexual problems around the time a woman goes through the menopause, but it is important to remember that this transition phase does not mark the end of a sexual relationship. Men also often experience a period of physiological and hormonal change, often referred to as a 'mid-life' crisis. Unfortunately, this can often occur while their partners are going through the menopause. Subsequently, many men make rash and ill-judged decisions during this time with devastating consequences, for example the break-up of a long and happy marriage or partnership.

Similarly, if men experience a problem, their partners should take time to consider its physiological nature. Older men in particular can take a little longer to obtain an erection. If a man's partner reacts to such problems by belittling his performance or making scornful remarks, this will greatly hinder any resolution of the situation. On the other hand, patience and gentle encouragement will be of benefit. Women can usually live without achieving orgasm, but men who do not achieve ejaculation suffer a great loss of self-esteem and believe that they may have a serious health problem. In such circumstances, the more a man's partner pressurises him into achieving ejaculation, the harder it will become for him to achieve satisfactory sexual function. Achieving this can be made much easier by help and understanding.

A sexual relationship is a joint activity that should give pleasure, enjoyment and satisfaction to both partners, and unhappiness can easily arise if one partner is not achieving any of these within a sexual relationship. Taking time to discuss and communicate each other's wants and desires can help to prevent such problems. For example, a woman will not enjoy or receive pleasure from sexual activity if she feels that her partner has 'forced' or co-erced' her into participating when she is feeling emotionally negative and unresponsive. Cold responses to sexual activity can wreck a partnership. If a couple are unable to discuss the problems that have arisen within their sexual relationship, professional outside advice should be sought.

Above all, a good sense of humour can play a major role in safeguarding the sanity of a marriage or partnership. A shared sense of humour goes a long way in making any relationship successful. Sexual problems are fairly common, and humour can help partners to break through the awkwardness that often accompanies such areas.

Sexual harmony, friendship, mutual understanding and a good sense of humour will give you the basis of a sound partnership enabling you to communicate with your partner and consequently maintain and strengthen a happy, loving relationship well into your later years, a good way indeed to ensure you feel fabulous.

15

How do I keep my brain active in retirement?

In the excellent magazine *Home and Life*, an interviewer talking to Gloria stated that she was one of today's most engaging television stars. Although we are both still working, Gloria and I have often discussed the subject of retirement. We both have very full lives – I still work ninety hours a week at the age of nearly sixty-three and Gloria nearly as many at a few years younger. Gloria is rightly proud of this achievement and says that keeping yourself interested in the world about you – maybe simply by ensuring that you read the newspaper every day – is crucial. I firmly believe that this interest in and enjoyment of life is the basis of anyone continuing to enjoy good health and vitality.

I find that I am at my most energetic when I have a daily schedule to get through. Gloria keeps active by enjoying her busy work schedule, as much as she enjoys her leisure time, and has never considered the possibility of retirement. It is possible that neither of us wishes to think of retiring but wants to continue enjoying the satisfaction of accomplishing a full day's work. We are also lucky enough to have jobs that do not force us to retire at sixty.

The best method of approaching 'retirement' is to keep the brain ticking over. We keep up to date on daily happenings, taking life as Gloria's father always used to say 'one day at a time'. We all wish to keep our minds active and alert: my grandmother was still mentally and physically active at the age of ninety-eight, claiming that the secret of enjoying old age is to keep up to date with all that is going on around you.

On the other hand, some people feel that they had had enough of work and look forward to retirement to do the things they have always wanted to. Others, forced to retire from their jobs, may take the chance to learn a new career or new skills. There are numerous options available – a wide range of sports and interests that can help to keep both the mind and body active. As we said in the chapter on exercise, mental exercise is just as important as physical in keeping us feeling fabulous. What is crucial is that we look on this time of our life – whether or not we are in paid work – as a challenge and full of excitement. This may also help and alleviate boredom and make those of us who feel we are no longer of any use to society realise that we still have a lot to give – to our communities, to our friends, and to ourselves as a reward.

Retirement is a great opportunity to evaluate your life. My wife decided to retire from her teaching position as she approached sixty as hers was not an easy job. I have noted with great interest her subsequent approach to life. She is certainly not the type of person to sit around and vegetate! My wife was always greatly interested in museums and she has kept this up; she is also a great reader. However, her main interest lay with animals, so she decided to keep a flock of sheep, not only for enjoyment, but also for study and research. As the years went by, she felt that she was putting on too much weight, and so she took up exercise, and in particular line-dancing, with great enthusiasm. She also undertook voluntary work for the Red Cross and developed her skills in spinning and weaving. My wife leads a very full and interesting life, and her retirement has certainly not led her to sitting around vegetating; nobody wants that.

We will know when the time has come to put the brakes on and to recognise that we have had enough of the daily routine. You will then wish to spend your time and effort on something that gives you enjoyment and satisfaction – with so many things to choose from. This strong desire is very understandable, especially if you have worked very hard all your life and wish to make the most of your retirement years. I greatly admire couples who adjust to retirement together and find their lives to be more fulfilling and satisfying than ever.

The other day I was asked to give a talk to an over-fifties group. In the middle of the talk, I stopped because I knew that I was talking to many people who were younger than me – perhaps I ought to be pensioned off! Realising that you are of a certain age is a good thing, but you have to be careful not to develop a phobia about getting old, then becoming obsessed with keeping young. One has to accept one's age and the differing opportunities that are available at different times during our lives. At the same time, however, one also has to take into account one's state of health: it is not advisable to undertake activities that are beyond one's current capacity.

I have often seen people approaching retirement who think that their worries are over and that all they have to do is sit back and relax. These people have no vision or imagination. Imagination is a very important element in attaining your goals and achieving satisfaction, especially for the over-fifties. People differ in imagination: some are said to have vivid imaginations, others none at all. The painter, recreating a new image composed of a number of elements from his experience, is giving practical expression to a combination of what he has seen. The novelist reshuffles his experience; his stories are combinations of what has happened to him, what he has read and what he has learned in conversation with others. The skill, or the degree of novelty, with which the painter or novelist constructs these new combinations shows the creative quality of his imagination.

How does our imagination collect all the information to work with? When you recall an experience, you do so in various ways. Suppose you recollect your first visit to a new friend's house. You may form mental images of what the garden looked like, how the house was furnished and so on. These are visual images. A memory of the scent of the flowers – *an image of smell* – may come to you, as may the soft feeling as you trod on the grass – *a tactile image* – or the noise of the traffic in the street – *an auditory image*, or the muscular effort involved in climbing up the stairs – *a motor image*. You will learn more about these different kinds of image on the following pages. The most common type of image, and the one which predominates with most people, is the *visual image*, although the other types are experienced by the majority of individuals at different times.

If a person recalls images based on past experience and recombines the various elements to produce a novel result, he is said to have a vivid imagination. You have had many moments in your life when your mind has formed and reformed images from the past. If this is done extensively during your waking hours, you will be called a day-dreamer. At night, when your body is resting, and you are asleep, past experiences flood back into your memory. The elements may be combined simply, or fantastically distorted, in what we call dreams.

Psychologists explain dreams partly by saying that they fulfil our wishes. The poor man dreams of possessing riches; the child dreams of the toys her parents cannot afford to buy her; the individual who, in real life, lacks the energy to achieve his ambition, dreams that he has done so. Thus, when you cannot get what you want in reality, you may seek satisfaction in dreams; you give the various elements in your mind a new direction, when you dream, until they are combined into the picture you want – with yourself in the centre.

If you do this consciously during your waking hours with a definite goal in mind, the result will be something new and useful. You are making proper use of your imagination. But if you allow yourself to create a dream picture simply because real life has denied what you desire, you begin to live falsely. You are in danger of finding so much satisfaction in your dream world that you become entirely divorced from the responsibilities of your real existence. You come to live in a world created by your imagination.

You have probably seen many new inventions that have made fortunes for those who had the imagination to think of them and the energy to apply what originally evolved as a mental image. Many brilliant inventors have failed to reap the benefit of their work because they have been only dreamers and have not been able to make practical use of their creations. Success demands a concrete application of what you have built up in your mind.

When a new idea has been explained, I am sure that you have often asked yourself why you did not think of it before. The reason may be that you have not had the essential experience or training. More probably, however, it is because your imagination has not been trained so that you are able to recombine the elements of your experience in the form necessary to produce the result that surprises you with its simplicity once you have seen how it has been done. New ideas are very often nothing more than a rearrangement of old experiences – possibly a complete reshuffling of elements, or perhaps only a minor addition to an existing combination.

It was because men with imagination saw birds flying in the air that they imagined they too could fly. If this had remained just a dream, without any effort being made to fulfil it, flight would never have been achieved. It was because energy, experience and scientific knowledge were brought to bear, to give practical expression to a dream, that aeroplanes were developed.

On the other hand, not every goal that the imagination presents is capable of attainment. Just because you are deeply interested in the theatre and love to picture yourself as a successful actor, it does not follow that you are therefore fitted for a lead role in an amateur dramatic company – but maybe you could get involved backstage or as a pair of hands in the box office. Imagination, to be a useful driving force, must be harnessed by the powers and abilities you really do possess.

Great talkers are seldom great doers. Think, then act, rather than talk as otherwise the chances are that all your energy will be expended in chatter. The person who describes at length what he is going to do is invariably merely another type of day-dreamer. Instead of obtaining satisfaction by doing something, he obtains all the reward he desires from only telling people what he intends to do. The man who achieves his goal rarely discusses his actions at length with anyone unless he has a definite purpose. He proceeds with calm, silent confidence, thinking instead of talking.

So let your imagination set for you the goal of what you want to achieve in your retirement; this will provide the incentive. Imagine yourself having achieved your object. Picture the advantages and the satisfaction you will enjoy. Without such a stimulus, your efforts will lack the dynamic force necessary to sustain them and bring them to a successful conclusion. Don't forget that you must act in addition to dreaming about acting. Control your imagination, so that all the powers within you are directed towards giving concrete expression to your ambitious dreams. Then you will succeed and nothing will hold you back.

Another factor that helps us to make the most of retirement is the ability to concentrate. This will enable your brain to function to its best. Training your concentration and memory will be discussed below. Using the preparation Memory Factors from Michael's (one tablet twice a day) can be of help, as can Dr Vogel's *Ginkgo biloba* or the flower essence Concentration Essence; all these are available from health food shops. Improving the concentration is a talent that must not be neglected.

Every moment of your life, whether you are asleep or awake, things are happening around you. The majority pass unnoticed, but a few are recorded in your mind, mostly temporarily, sometimes permanently. Have you ever paused to consider how far you really are aware of everything that is occurring? Why do you become conscious of certain people and certain objects, yet remain quite unconscious of others?

The reason is that the capacity of your mind for absorbing impressions from the outside world is limited. If the greatest use is to be made of this capacity, it is important that you should select those items from your everyday life to which it will be most useful for you to devote your attention. Unfortunately, it is not always possible to do this. Certain experiences, by reason of their vividness or intensity, force themselves into your field of attention, to the exclusion of everything else. Abnormally loud noises, bright colours and unusual occurrences compel you to attend to them. But you can control your attention and concentrate upon work which you need to do, people and objects you are interested in and want to know more about, and so on.

You have probably known moments when your mind is a complete blank, when everything around you is a confused blur. Such a period is called dispersed attention. Suddenly, you rouse yourself, attention becomes concentrated upon a single object, and life begins to move forward again. This is concentrated attention, your mind being so absorbed in the interest of the moment that you are oblivious to everything else. At tense moments during a football match, spectators forget the discomfort of being in a crowd, the rain that may be falling, everything except the actions of the men on the field.

Dispersed attention is also seen when you attempt to deal with several things at once, for example watching the on-coming traffic while crossing a road and at the same time observing two dogs fighting on the opposite pavement. Neither the traffic nor the dogs will receive your complete attention, with possibly unfortunate results. While we are learning a new task, we must use concentrated attention. For example, a woman cannot concentrate effectively upon learning to knit while she is carrying on a conversation. If she tries this, neither activity will be performed properly. But if one activity is reduced to a habit, her attention is free for the effective performance of the other: once she has learnt to knit, it will no longer be essential to concentrate upon each stitch.

The immature, underdeveloped mind is at the mercy of everything that intrudes upon it. The child notices the loudest noise, the brightest colour – any stimulus that has an exciting quality. Her attention drifts from one object to another. The mature mind selects as the objects of attention those happenings which are related to permanent interests and purposes, and excludes all others. To do this requires training – the cultivation of the habit of controlling the direction of attention, involving a rigorous exclusion of all irrelevant distractions from the field of consciousness. When you reach this stage, you become the master of yourself rather than the slave of your environment. Your mind belongs to you, not to every object that happens to catch your attention.

Voluntary attention requires effort, which will vary according to the interest you find in the material on which you want to concentrate, and the intensity of other distractions. It is most difficult to concentrate upon things that have no meaning or no relation to your needs and interests. Concentration is made easier if you discover meaning and interest in what you do. Your attention continually wanders from that which is meaningless, so make a point of finding out the implications of everything you do, and then the effort of attending will be diminished and your task will be better achieved.

As we have said, voluntary attention becomes more difficult if your *in*voluntary attention is being continually excited by your surroundings. Concentrating on a mathematical problem is difficult if someone is talking to you, if the radio or television is on, or if a multitude of other excitements are clamouring for your attention. Writing a letter becomes an effort if your pen is scratching or the light is bad. So give yourself a chance to concentrate. Do not handicap yourself by tolerating an environment full of minor and unnecessary distractions. They can nearly always be removed without difficulty: the scratching pen must be replaced, the bad light improved, the noise shut out, and so on.

Bodily states, too, may impede concentration. A healthy body, free from ills and pains, is a valuable aid to controlled attention, as is a mind that is kept clear of fears, inferiority feelings and other such factors. It is obviously very difficult to concentrate if some emotional conflict is dividing the mind. This may be particularly relevant as you learn to be retired as you may be feeling less than confident in such a new situation.

Certain times of the day are also more favourable for concentration than others, although these tend to vary between individuals. In general, the early morning is better than late at night, and it is a good plan, when possible, to get the most difficult tasks done before noon.

Voluntary attention can be greatly strengthened by training yourself to observe accurately because, in order to observe, you must pay attention. You may think that little escapes your notice, but tests show that it is remarkable how little is noticed by most people. Police officers, for example, have the greatest difficulty in obtaining reliable descriptions of wanted felons. Can *you* say with assurance the colour of the eyes of even your closest friends?

If you have difficulty in training your attention on any subject you wish, give yourself practice in observation every day. Try and fix in your mind the order and types of the shops in your nearest high street. Make a point of noticing the distinctive mannerisms of your friends. Make yourself observe the colour of their eyes and hair, the shape of their hands and nails.

You will soon find that your interest is aroused, and your powers of attention will automatically grow. From time to time, give yourself the following test. Ask a friend to cover a small table with a number of miscellaneous objects – a penknife, a cigarette case, a reel of cotton, a pair of gloves, for example. Look at the table for a given period of time – say five, ten or fifteen seconds. Go away and write down everything you saw on the table. This will serve to test your observation and train your memory at the same time.

Let us now consider how you might train yourself to attend to some daily routine task that you find difficult in carrying out because your thoughts continually wander to other matters.

First, discover an interest in your task, deriving this interest from whatever result is attached to it. If something you are called upon to do does not immediately awaken your curiosity, you must create an interest. Take the most boring part of your work, on which up till now you have found it difficult to concentrate. Strive to understand the significance of your duties, find meaning in them, and concentrating will be made easier.

Here is another exercise in concentration. You may be troubled by an incapacity to absorb a difficult passage you are reading, or unable to concentrate upon complicated instructions. It will be easier to keep your attention from wandering if you echo the words in your mind or even read it out loud. Tomorrow, when you read the leading article in your daily paper, try this method, and discover how it helps you ignore other distractions; the meaning will become more quickly apparent to you and you will concentrate more easily.

There are three components of memory:

- attention, involving concentration upon the experience registered in the mind, which we have considered above
- retention, or the process of mental registration, so that the experience can be recalled – see below for more on this
- recall, or recollection

Let us consider the process of recall in more detail. How do we recollect? How do we train ourselves to recall relevant experiences at the right time? How do we act in relation to events we know we must remember at definite times in the future?

In training your capacity for recollection at an appropriate moment, you must form an association between the mental image of what is to be remembered and another image or experience that you know will occur at the time when you wish the recollection to take place.

For example, a wife may ask her husband to bring home a bunch of flowers to brighten up the dining room. He may follow the age-old tradition of tying a piece of string around his little finger so that he does not forget. He associates the idea of bringing home the flowers with the string on his finger. Each time he sees string on his finger during the day, he will make the mental link between it and the flowers.

Recollection is thus dependent upon the mental association of one event or object with others, and the effectiveness with which you create these associations will determine the effectiveness of your recollection.

Some minds are naturally like jelly that yields to any pressure but retains a permanent impression only with difficulty; other minds are capable of retaining everything once it has been experienced. Minds differ in their natural retentiveness, both between individuals and in the same individual at various stages of his or her life, and recollection is correspondingly affected. Those whose experiences, once they have been selected, stick in their minds are the ones who will progress. Others, whose minds, either naturally or through lack of training, are not so retentive often spend a considerable part of their time relearning what they have forgotten.

Here are a few more exercises to help to polish up your memory. As a beginning to training your memory, take a picture in your daily newspaper. Study it for half a minute and then put it to one side. Recall and write down what you have seen. You will find that the more meaning you are able to read into the picture, the more complete will be your ability to recall every detail.

Take a paragraph of printed matter, slowly read it over once and then try to write it out. Again, the more you have been able to systematise the material and give it meaning, the more you will remember.

Take a short poem that appeals to you and read it over carefully three or four times, making sure that you have grasped the succession of ideas and pictures it presents. Then put the book away and see how much of the poem you can repeat. In doing this exercise, you are advised to learn the whole poem at one time. Experiments have shown that it is easier to grasp and retain a sequence of thought than to remember isolated lines or phrases in their correct order. If you grasp the meaning, it will be easier to remember the words that express the meaning.

Finally, if your memory does not improve as rapidly as you would like, or if it is a constant source of weakness, let a properly kept diary and appointment pad do its work for you. You must be rigidly systematic in this matter. Enter every appointment as it is made; list your duties every day and cross off each one as it is fulfilled; note down telephone numbers and addresses in their proper place as soon as you learn them.

If your mind is not naturally retentive, you must also compensate for this disability by concentrating more upon connecting your selected experiences by association with your experience as a whole. The more you think over the experiences you wish to remember, the more they will become woven into associations with each other, and so the greater will be the ease with which you will recall the other.

Associations connected with your interests are the most easily formed. If you are interested in cricket, your ability to recollect dates in English history may be poor, but you will be able to retell to your friends the performances of outstanding players during the season. If your business interests are related to, say, radio, you will be able to remember an extraordinary number of facts about radio stations and presenters owing to the amount you have to think about them. On the other hand, you may not be able to recall the name of a single racehorse, just because your interests do not lie in that direction.

As described above in relation to imagination, the images or experiences recalled may be divided into five types: visual, tactile, auditory, smell and motor. One type of image frequently recalls another. You may associate specific scents with certain flowers: the sight of a hyacinth may recall to you a mental image of one odour, jasmine another. When you pass the Albert Hall, you may recollect music you once heard at a concert there. The more of these combinations of associations you form in your mind in connection with an experience, the more permanent will be your capacity for recollecting it. If you register in your mind what anything looks, feels, sounds and smells like, you will be able to recall it more easily than if you only register what it looks like.

Suppose, for example, on your last summer holiday, your mind was impressed by the warmth of the sun, the touch of the water on your skin, the smell of the sea, the sounds of children playing on the sands and the wonderful feeling of swimming and walking. Six months later, any chance reminder to any one of these senses will evoke the whole scene before you. If you only registered what the place looked like, you would be much less likely to remember it afterwards.

The wisest and most effective way of improving your memory is by developing your habitual method of registering facts in your mind. Repetition is the most commonly employed procedure, just like we all learned poetry at school by repeating it over and over again. Another is by intensifying the experience so that your attention must be concentrated upon it. In books, items that need to be remembered may be underlined, printed in large letters or set in bold type. These may be described as the mechanical methods or memorising.

In addition to the purely mechanical methods of memorising, the systematic method is that which attaches meaning to experiences, analysing and classifying them into systems. Words that have a meaning for you are more easily remembered than those which have none. If you form words into sentences to jog your memory, make them have a rhythmic association with each other, as in poetry, which makes them easier to memorise.

I am sure that you have been introduced to someone whose name you have later forgotten even though you can recognise their face on another meeting. The reason for this is that you have failed to form in your mind an association between the visual image of what the person looks like, and the oral image of his or her name, so that one spontaneously recalls the other. You can strengthen the associative link at a time when the introduction is made by concentrating upon forming as many associations as possible between the name, the oral image, and the facial characteristics or visual image. A man may, for example, be introduced to you as Mr Brown. He may have brown eyes, brown hair and brown skin, so associate these characteristics with his name. Then, when you see him again, the visual and oral images will be recalled simultaneously. Other names may not be so easy, but, with a little inventiveness, associations should be possible.

Suppose you are introduced to a Mr Blenkinsop. You note that he has blue eyes. *Bl*ue and *Bl*enkinsop both start with the same letters, so once you have formed this association, it will be easier to associate the image of his face with his name. In other words, whenever you wish to register in your mind two images so that they will be recalled together in the future, concentrate upon finding a common link that will associate them – inseparably tie them together.

In trying to recall, you should always give yourself a fair chance. Remember that you will do better when feeling confident and in good health than when you are depressed and tired. So, if you have to make a special effort of memory, see that you are in good condition for it.

At the same time, there are various other ways in which you can coax your mind to work. A modern psychologist has written: 'Look squarely at the person whose name you wish to recall, avoid doubts as to your ability to recall it; for doubt is itself a distraction. Put yourself back into the time when you formerly used this person's name.' Sometimes it is not easy to recall what you feel you ought to know perfectly well; it is on the tip of the tongue but you cannot quite remember. The correct method at such a time is not to hurry the mind but to wait for a minute or two. Such a pause often helps to recall what you want to know in a way that an active search does not.

There are a number of hindrances to recall: emotional disturbances, especially fear, check it. You see this particularly with stage fright. Many a speaker with a splendid outline of his speech and a number of clever epigrams in mind finds that fright obliterates these, and he has to sit down knowing that the best parts of his speech have been left unspoken. The only effective remedy against such a difficulty is knowledge of how to keep your emotions in check so that they do not swamp your mind. It is true that many systems have been devised to help memorising and these are, in some cases and to a certain extent, undoubtedly useful. But it has been said that whoever relies upon a complicated memory system resembles a tightrope walker so intent upon keeping his equilibrium as to be unable to attend to anything else. So as with so many other things, simple is beautiful.

When we do master improving our memory and concentration, we will be reminded of the paradox of Victor Hugo who was certainly a master of concentration when he wrote the following:

> There is neither fog nor problem in algebra
> Which can withstand, in the depths of the numbers or the skies
> The calm and intense fixation of the eyes.

The day when we come to grasp the power of concentration, we resemble a child who, playing with a lens, accidentally holds it towards the rays of the sun. She then discovers that, under the influence of the lens, the rays converge towards a point, and that if in the focus there lies a fragment of straw, this, to the child's amazement, bursts into flame. We, too, can be as amazed when we discover that, passing through the lens of concentration, thought becomes power.

During retirement, the ageing process – which really begins at birth – is very difficult to assess. Some people's condition rapidly deteriorates, possibly unrelated to the stresses of life. Others, however, manage to look and feel relatively young. This is often the result of keeping one's mind fresh and active; it is often a question of concentration and vitality.

Retirement often affects two, rather than one person. I have often see the situation in retirement when one partner, who has always enjoyed the run of the house, now finds he or she has to share with somebody else; conflict can then become as natural as breathing. In such circumstances there has to be a period of transition in which both partners adjust to being around each other for the majority for the day. It is here that a positive change will not be automatic; it will take time, understanding and patience. I have seen many couples in a situation of permanent conflict, not understanding each other, even after so many changes and adjustments were needed on both sides to try to regain harmony.

Within a relationship, the concept of perfection that we so often strive for is not necessary to understand each other's wants and needs. A relationship depends on what you have in common with each other, and not one of us is perfect. We continually look back and reflect on other's people's attitudes and emotions, seeing only what to us is perfection. If we look for perfection in ourselves, however, we will understand why everybody else is perfect in his or her own way.

When we can see that someone else is less than perfect, and can recognise our own imperfections, we should be grateful for common experiences. We should take each other in love, even in retirement, when we are so much together. Unconditional love, which is the practice of forgiveness, is important. It is also important that we remain aware of when we do not forgive, and we should strengthen our resolve to forgive others. Each one of us is entitled to forgiveness, and I can say this because I have often heard from older patients that they have fallen into a routine of continuing fighting and battling as they no longer understand each other. This battleground of conflict becomes a habit and they feel lost without the fighting. This is not the best way to enjoy retirement. Get out in the fresh air, swim together, walk together, make sure that your last years together are more joyful and fulfilling than your first.

Many problems like this that arise in retirement will benefit from looking forward rather than back, sharpening your mind to overcome freedom rather than routine, learn how to improve your health and combat fears of illness, meet new people and keep up with old colleagues whom you may miss. Although we cannot avoid all the ills of life, a positive attitude can help us to overcome and learn from them. Keeping your memory and concentration sharp will mean that you play an active part in life rather than sit and watch as a spectator on the sidelines.

But to will yourself to make the effort to learn to get involved, you need a positive attitude to life, and this we will cover in our final chapter.

16

How do I get the best out of life?

When we talked about energy in a previous chapter, we discussed positive and negative, as in the poles of a battery. In our attitudes, positive thought will always overcome negative, as the stronger of the two will always win. When negative thoughts overtake and one replaces that with a positive thought, the results are remarkable. Maintaining a positive attitude is the key to our mental progress forwards, just as food is the key to keeping our bodies healthy. A positive attitude makes one happy, it makes one feel good and optimistic, even fabulous. Examine your inner qualities and talents and tell yourself that you are beautiful, and you will be on the way to boosting your positive attitude.

We just have to look at the many ways by which positive action always wins over negative thought. It is therefore important that we know how energy works. We have only just scraped the surface in this book, but from the little we know and from the actions we take, it is important that we study it. Willpower is very important and is not needed in huge quantities. It is there when you need a firm mental image of what you want from a situation. You want to feel great and feel fabulous, so you will need the willpower to visualise the future.

I previously said that habits could often rule a life and that good habits are important. It is vital to create willpower by training our minds. Health, too, will depend on self-control. These aspects are connected with passions and emotions, and also with the motives they control. The will to have a positive attitude depends on the incentive that one is given: if interest is lacking, you will get nowhere. Try to work on something that you really do not like doing, such as having a cold bath or shower, or going for a walk, or even writing a letter, and you will find that your willpower will improve and create a much more positive attitude.

When the mind goes blank and everything blurs, however, concentrating on a positive attitude is not easy. Remember that positive is always stronger than negative, and with a positive attitude, tasks will become much less of a burden. An immature, undeveloped mind is at the mercy of everything that intrudes, whereas a mature mind selects the objects of attention and excludes all others. This requires training, but you can learn to direct your thoughts. You are the one who is in control. The previous chapter gives you lots of information on how to train your memory and concentration to do this.

We all look for happiness in life and will probably find it with a positive attitude. Happiness can be hidden inaccessibly, but is there to be found in our own everyday lives. Everyone can be to some extent, successful and happy; how happy and successful we are is largely up to us. As part of this, we need to ask ourselves from time to time: 'Have I discovered my real self, and can I plan my life with a practical and positive attitude?' 'Have I overcome my fears, worries and selfish thoughts?' 'Are my habits good enough to please my partner?' 'Am I fit and healthy?' 'Is my attitude towards sexual matters positive?' 'Am I successful in what I do?' We must come to the conclusion that, in order to get the right answers, we have to do something about it now. It is never too late, but it is certainly better to act sooner rather than later.

I remember a listener from one of Gloria's programmes who wrote to me. She said that she felt that she was the most miserable, wretched and fed-up creature on earth. She was past fifty and no longer felt attractive. Her husband had run off with a younger woman, and she believed that her life had ended. She said that, while listening to one of our programmes, she looked in the mirror and saw all her wrinkles, leaving her feeling further depressed. She had heard me on the radio encouraging others, and she wanted to know what on earth there was left for her to live for.

At the time, I had a clinic in Birmingham, where this woman lived, so I wrote back to her and suggested that she come along and see me. This she did. She turned up describing herself as 'that old, cantankerous woman'. I looked at her carefully and noted immediately her lovely, brown eyes and her beautiful thick and wavy hair, which had very little grey in it. I said, 'Okay, you have some wrinkles and crows feet, and I shall help to smooth these out for you. However, in return I ask that you use your sense of humour. You need to learn to enjoy your life again. I will give you acupuncture to help lessen the wrinkles. I can also give you other treatments to help you feel younger and improve your health. I am sure that with my treatment and your own efforts, we will be able to turn you inside out and totally reverse your current attitude.'

One year later, this lady married a doctor who adores her. To this day, I continue to receive letters saying that she fervently believes she is now the happiest woman in the world. All is took was a positive attitude, followed by some positive action, to get where she wanted to be.

I recently saw a patient whom I wrote about in my book *Inner Harmony*. He went bankrupt because three people deceived him, then lost his only daughter and next came home to find a note from his wife telling him she had left him, taking most of the furniture with her. The only true friend he had, his dog, died. He said to me, 'How can I keep a positive attitude?' I encouraged him by saying, 'You still have your two hands, you still have your brain; try to start again.' When I saw him recently with his new partner, he seemed to be the happiest man in the world. A whole new life had opened because he faced up to it with a positive attitude; he even found that he was a lot happier with his new partner than he had been with his wife.

The way is not always smooth and there are often difficulties. It is often said that adversity makes us stronger and allows characteristics to develop that were previously unknown to us. It sometimes helps to look at other people and see how they confront problems and overcome their difficulties. Difficulties can be faced if we have a positive attitude and even though we might feel we lose everything, we still have ourselves and the challenge to start again to make a better life.

When I was dictating this chapter, I was sitting on a train from Glasgow to Preston; in the next set of seats was a lady who was very well dressed and made-up but had great difficulty in walking. I admired the beautiful smile on her face and couldn't help talking to her. She told me that she had multiple sclerosis, which caused her great difficulty in moving. 'I have done everything possible,' she said. 'I have kept myself mobile up to a point while some friends have ended up in wheelchairs. I do everything I can to keep mobile, and my mind is stronger than my body because I want to keep being positive. Because of my positive attitude I can face the world with a smile.' This lady did not sit back and let herself go. She was nicely dressed, was well make-up and had a very beautiful aura that also attracted some of my fellow passengers. In my little corner where I dictated this chapter, I looked at her and thought of many of my patients who were probably in the depths of despair, yet had the same or better opportunities than this lady. Being positive and keeping an active mind will encourage a positive attitude so you can get the most out of what you have.

I also recall a fellow student who had many struggles in life and no money from his parents to help him with his study, yet he had a goal. He was not the most intelligent person in the class but he had a positive attitude to everything. In sports, in his schooling, in his life, he wanted to get on. He worked in the evenings, and when I later met him again, he had become managing director of one of the biggest companies in Holland, all because of his positive attitude. A positive attitude always wins.

This is a bit like the story of the old man of ninety-nine who went to his shoemaker. The shoemaker said to him, 'Why are you so fussy and impatient about this pair of shoes: you are ninety-nine, do you think you are going to live to wear them out?' The old man was very angry and replied, 'My good man, don't you realise that few people die at the age of ninety-nine. Statistics prove it.'

So as we get older, we want to become younger, we want to look fabulous. When I looked at my old partner, Dr Vogel, who was still skiing at the age of ninety-seven, he still looked like a young man. I look at all my old friends who took a little lesson from nature and did what nature told them to do; they too kept young. We obviously cannot neglect our bodies; what we put into them, they will try to give back to us. But the mind is stronger than the body, and a positive attitude will help to pave the way for that youthful look that we all want to maintain. It is much better to be a happy, healthy person of fifty than a weak imitation of one of twenty. Nobody really admires a person who tries to hide their age from themselves and others. Plan to be a marvel for your age as you grow older, but do not try to remain a marvel for some age that has passed you by. The secret of being a marvel for your age is a positive attitude. And don't lose your interest in life as it is this which keeps you young.

When I look at Gloria, with whom I do so many radios and television broadcasts, she still jumps around like a twenty-year-old, has this fantastic positive attitude and can do more now than she could when she *was* twenty. Time and experience have built your character and personality into that of the person you are today. Whether this has occurred for twenty or forty years or more, the point is that you have been interested in life and want to make it better still. It is the positive attitude that underlies our happiness to adapt and live life to the full now.

Plato, in *The Republic*, said:

> What is the prime of Life? May it not be defined as a period of about twenty years in a woman's life and thirty in a man's life.

After you have read this book, I hope that you will be equipped to prove Plato wrong, showing that all of us over fifty can look and feel fabulous for many years to come.

Suppliers

Most of the products mentioned in the book, as well as many other suitable and effective products, can be obtained from chemists and health food shops. If there is any problem, the manufacturer can be contacted directly.

Bioforce
Irvine
Ayrshire
KA11 5DD

HHC
Freepost
Hadley Wood
Barnet
Hertfordshire
EN4 0EJ

Lamberts/Nature's Best
PO Box 1
Tunbridge Wells
Kent
TN2 3EQ

SHP
Troon
Ayrshire
KA10 7EL

Bibliography

Baudoin, C., *The Power Within Us* (George Allan).
Bremer, S., *Health, Wealth and Happiness* (Successful Achievement).
Brown, H. and Walker, P., *Breezing Through the Change* (Walker).
Campion, K., *Holistic Womans Herbal* (Live Successfully).
Cherry, S. H., *The Woman's Guide to Health* (Granada).
Clark, J., *Bodyfoods For Women* (Wiedenfield & Nicholson).
Dalet, R., *Relief from Pain with Finger Massage* (Hutchinson).
De Marco, C., *The Charge of Your Body* (Wellwoman Press).
Devi, I., *Forever Young, Forever Healthy* (Morrison & Gibb).
de Vries, J., *Body Energy* (Mainstream).
de Vries, J., *Nature's Gift of Food* (Mainstream).
de Vries, J., *Menopause* (Mainstream).
de Vries, J., *Stress and Nervous Disorders* (Mainstream).
de Vries, J., *Inner Harmony* (Mainstream).
Dowden, A. and Lacey, G., *The Consumer Guide to Vitamins* (Macmillan).
Karslow, A. and Miles, R., *You Can Achieve Freedom of Chronic Disease* (JP Publishing).

Lark, S. M., *The Menopause Self Help Book* (Celestial Arts).
Melville, A., *Natural Hormone Health* (Thorsons).
Oddenino, K., *Sharing: The Self-discovery in a Relationship* (Joy Publications).
Shapiro, D., *The Bodywork Book* (Element Books).
Shreeve, C. M., *Overcoming Menopause Naturally* (Arrow Books).
Valins, L., *Intimate Matters* (Gaia).
Vogel, A., *The Nature Doctor* (A. Vogel Verlag).
Webb, M. and Webb, M., *Healing Touch* (Godsfield Press).